A POCKET MANUAL OF DIFFERENTIAL DIAGNOSIS

Second Edition

Stephen N. Adler, M.D.
Clinical Instructor in Medicine, University of Oklahoma
College of Medicine; Medical Director, Respiratory Therapy,
Mercy Health Center, Oklahoma City

Mildred Lam, M.D.
Assistant Professor of Medicine, Case Western Reserve
University School of Medicine; Assistant Director,
Hemodialysis Unit, Nephrology Division, Cleveland
Metropolitan General Hospital, Cleveland

Dianne B. Gasbarra, M.D.
Clinical Instructor in Medicine, University of Oklahoma
College of Medicine; Internist and Pulmonary Disease
Specialist, Mercy Health Center, Oklahoma City

Alfred F. Connors, Jr., M.D.
Assistant Professor of Medicine, Case Western Reserve
University School of Medicine; Director, Medical Intensive
Care Unit, Pulmonary Disease and Critical Care Division,
Cleveland Metropolitan General Hospital, Cleveland

Little, Brown and Company
Boston/Toronto

To Our Parents

CONTENTS

3. Drugs 57
Stephen N. Adler

4. Endocrine/Metabolic System 87
Thomas A. Murphy

13. Respiratory System 303
Alfred F. Connors, Jr.

CONTRIBUTING AUTHORS

David J. Adelstein, M.D.
Assistant Professor of Medicine, Case Western Reserve University
School of Medicine; Associate Director, Hematology-Oncology
Division, Cleveland Metropolitan General Hospital, Cleveland

Stephen N. Adler, M.D.
Clinical Instructor in Medicine, University of Oklahoma College of
Medicine; Medical Director, Respiratory Therapy, Mercy Health
Center, Oklahoma City

Bruce R. Bacon, M.D.
Associate Professor of Medicine and Physiology & Biophysics,
Louisiana State University School of Medicine in Shreveport; Chief,
Section of Gastroenterology, Louisiana State University Medical
Center, Shreveport

Alfred F. Connors, Jr., M.D.
Assistant Professor of Medicine, Case Western Reserve University
School of Medicine; Director, Medical Intensive Care Unit, Pulmonary
Disease and Critical Care Division, Cleveland Metropolitan General
Hospital, Cleveland

Dianne B. Gasbarra, M.D.
Clinical Instructor in Medicine, University of Oklahoma College of
Medicine; Internist and Pulmonary Disease Specialist, Mercy Health
Center, Oklahoma City

Mildred Lam, M.D.
Assistant Professor of Medicine, Case Western Reserve University
School of Medicine; Assistant Director, Hemodialysis Unit,
Nephrology Division, Cleveland Metropolitan General Hospital,
Cleveland

Thomas A. Murphy, M.D.
Assistant Professor of Medicine, Case Western Reserve University
School of Medicine; Director, Endocrinology Division, Cleveland
Metropolitan General Hospital, Cleveland

PREFACE

In the practice of clinical medicine, one encounters a variety of symptoms, signs, and laboratory tests. Each clinical finding and test result is associated with a differential diagnosis, i.e., a list of conditions or disease entities that can produce the given finding or result. Differential diagnoses for various clinical findings are readily available in medical texts and other sources, but the information is often scattered in a number of different references. Our book contains information that has been gathered from many such sources and has been compiled in a compact form. It therefore serves as a convenient guide in the workup of clinical problems and is valuable as a teaching tool as well. Intended for the use of medical students, physician's assistants, house officers, and practicing and teaching clinicians, this book can help to make the process of medical diagnosis more efficient and comprehensive. It does not, however, serve as a substitute for the thoughtful, skillful integration of data obtained by careful history-taking, physical examination, and judicious use of laboratory tests.

The new edition, like the first, is divided into 13 sections: ten organ systems, and sections on acid-base/electrolyte disorders, drugs, and infectious diseases. Each section contains multiple entries, which represent symptoms, clinical signs, laboratory tests, radiologic findings, and disease processes; there is a total of 189 entries. The differential diagnosis for each entry is listed, with more common disease

entities generally being listed first; extremely rare entities
or those of questionable documentation are often omitted.
Where possible, disease entities are organized by pathophysiologic mechanism. At the end of each entry, a number
of references, usually general or subspecialty texts, are
listed. Entries are cross-referenced, and the book is indexed. A bibliography of general and subspecialty texts is
also included at the end of the book.

We acknowledge the expert secretarial assistance of
Fran Apltauer, Pat Garnett, Connie Jones, Anne LaGania,
and Joan Skiba. We are also grateful to our editors, Susan
Pioli and Katherine Arnoldi of Little, Brown, who helped to
prepare this edition. Finally, we would like to give special
acknowledgment to the housestaff and medical students of
the Case Western Reserve medical community, whose
support and encouragement have made it worthwhile to
prepare the second edition of this book.

S.N.A.
M.L.
D.B.G.
A.F.C.

A POCKET
MANUAL OF
DIFFERENTIAL
DIAGNOSIS

Notice

The indications and dosages of all drugs in this book have been recommended in the medical literature and conform to the practices of the general medical community. The medications described do not necessarily have specific approval by the Food and Drug Administration for use in the diseases and dosages for which they are recommended. The package insert for each drug should be consulted for use and dosage as approved by the FDA. Because standards for usage change, it is advisable to keep abreast of revised recommendations, particularly those concerning new drugs.

1 ACID-BASE AND ELECTROLYTE DISORDERS

1-A. Acid-Base Nomogram

Source: Goldberg M, Green SB, Moss ML, et al: Computer-Based Instruction and Diagnosis of Acid-Base Disorders. *JAMA* 223:270, 1973. Copyright © 1973 by the American Medical Association.

1-B. Metabolic Acidosis

Increased Anion Gap
Renal failure, acute or chronic
Ketoacidosis
   Diabetic
   Alcoholic
   Starvation
Lactic acidosis (see 1-E)
Toxins
   Aspirin
   Methanol
   Ethylene glycol
   Paraldehyde
   Toluene
Nonketotic hyperosmolar coma
Inborn errors of metabolism (e.g., maple syrup urine disease, methylmalonic aciduria)

Normal Anion Gap
Gastrointestinal loss
   Diarrhea
   Ileal loop, ureterosigmoidostomy
   Small-bowel or pancreatic fistula or drainage
   Anion-exchange resins (e.g., cholestyramine)
   Calcium or magnesium chloride ingestion
Renal loss
   Renal tubular acidosis (see 7-F)
   Hypoaldosteronism
   Carbonic anhydrase inhibitors
Recovery phase of ketoacidosis
Rapid expansion of extracellular fluid volume with bicarbonate-free fluid
Hyperalimentation with excess of cationic amino acids
Acidifying agents (e.g., ammonium chloride, arginine hydrochloride, lysine hydrochloride)
Sulfur ingestion

References
1. Kaehny WD, Gabow PA: Pathogenesis and Management of Metabolic Acidosis and Alkalosis. In general reference 16, p 141.
2. Narins RG, Krishna GG, Bressler L: The Metabolic Acidoses. In general reference 6, p 597.

1-C. Respiratory Acidosis

Neuromuscular Causes
Ingestion or overdose (e.g., tranquilizers, sedatives, anes-
  thetics, anticholinesterases)
Cerebral, brainstem, or high spinal-cord injury or infarct
Primary neuromuscular disease
  Guillain-Barré syndrome
  Myasthenia gravis
  Amyotrophic lateral sclerosis
  ...myelitis
  Botulism
  Tetanus
Myopathy involving respiratory muscles, especially:
  Muscular dystrophy
  Hypokalemic myopathy
  Familial periodic paralysis
Primary hypoventilation
Sleep apnea syndrome
Diaphragmatic paralysis

Airway Obstruction
Upper airway
  Laryngeal edema or spasm
  Tracheal edema, stenosis
  Obstructive sleep apnea
Lower airway
  Mechanical
    Foreign body
    Aspirated fluid (e.g., vomitus)
    Neoplasm
  Bronchospasm
    Acute
    Chronic (chronic obstructive pulmonary disease)

Cardiopulmonary-Thoracic Causes
Cardiac arrest
Severe pneumonia
Severe pulmonary edema
Respiratory distress syndrome (infant or adult)
Restrictive lung disease (e.g., interstitial fibrosis)
Massive pulmonary embolism
Pneumothorax, hemothorax
Chest trauma
Kyphoscoliosis
Smoke inhalation
Improper mechanical ventilation

References
1. Gennari FJ: Respiratory Acidosis and Alkalosis. In general reference 6, p 713.
2. Kaehny WD: Pathogenesis and Management of Respiratory and Mixed Acid-Base Disorders. In general reference 16, p 187.

1-D. Anion Gap

Increased
Without acidosis
  Administration of sodium salts of organic compounds
    (e.g., citrate, lactate, acetate)
  High-dose penicillin or carbenicillin
  Respiratory or metabolic alkalosis
  Dehydration
With acidosis
  Renal failure, acute or chronic
  Ketoacidosis
    Diabetic
    Starvation
    Alcoholic
  Nonketotic hyperosmolar coma
  Lactic acidosis (see 1-E)
  Toxins
    Aspirin
    Methanol
    Ethylene glycol
    Paraldehyde
    Toluene
  Inborn errors of metabolism

Decreased
Hypoalbuminemia
Hypernatremia, severe
Dilution of extracellular fluid
Multiple myeloma
Hyperviscosity
Bromide ingestion
Hypercalcemia, hypermagnesemia (severe)
Lithium toxicity

References
1. Emmett M, Narins RG: Clinical Use of the Anion Gap. *Medicine* 56:38, 1977.
2. Oh MS, Carroll HJ: Current Concepts: The Anion Gap. *N Engl J Med* 297:814, 1977.

1-E. Lactic Acidosis

Associated with Impaired Tissue Oxygenation (Type A)

Shock (e.g., hypovolemic, cardiogenic, septic)
Hypoxemia, respiratory failure
Anemia, severe

Occurring in Absence of Apparent Hypoxemia or Circulatory Insufficiency (Type B)

Diabetes, uncontrolled
Hepatic failure
Renal failure
Malignancy, especially leukemia or lymphoma
Drugs, toxins
   Cyanide
   Carbon monoxide
   Methanol
   Salicylates
   Iron
   Strychnine
   Ethanol
Seizures
Excessive muscular activity (e.g., excessive exercise)
Alkalosis, respiratory or metabolic
D-Lactic acidosis (secondary to intestinal bacterial overgrowth)
Congenital enzyme deficiency (e.g, glycogen storage disease)

References
1. Kaehny WD, Gabow PA: Pathogenesis and Management of Metabolic Acidosis and Alkalosis. In general reference 16, p 141.
2. Narins RG, Krishhna GG, Bressler L, et al: The Metabolic Acidoses. In general reference 6, p 597.
3. Kreisberg RA: Lactate Homeostasis and Lactic Acidosis. *Ann Intern Med* 92:227, 1980.

1-F. Metabolic Alkalosis

Chloride-Responsive (Urine Cl^- < 10 mEq/L)
Vomiting, nasogastric suction
Gastric drainage or fistula
Diuretics
Posthypercapnic state
Villous adenoma of colon
Congenital chloride diarrhea
Cystic fibrosis

Chloride-Resistant (Urine Cl^- > 20 mEq/L)
Primary aldosteronism
Secondary aldosteronism
  Congestive heart failure
  Cirrhosis and ascites
  Malignant hypertension
  Adrenocorticotropic hormone (ACTH) or glucocorticoid
    excess (Cushing's disease, Cushing's syndrome, ec-
    topic ACTH production)
  Bartter's syndrome
  Renin-secreting tumor (e.g., hemangiopericytoma)
Licorice ingestion
Excessive use of chewing tobacco
Severe potassium depletion
Congenital adrenal hyperplasia
Liddle's syndrome

Miscellaneous
Administration of alkali or alkalinizing agents, especially in
    the presence of renal insufficiency:
  Alkalinizing agents (e.g., citrate, lactate)
  Antacids (milk-alkali syndrome)
  Massive transfusion of blood or plasma substitute
Nonparathyroid hypercalcemia (e.g., bone metastases,
    multiple myeloma)
Nonreabsorbable anionic antibiotics, large doses (e.g.,
    penicillin, carbenicillin)
Glucose ingestion after starvation

References
1. Kaehny WD, Gabow PA: Pathogenesis and Management
   of Metabolic Acidosis and Alkalosis. In general reference
   16, p 141.
2. Sabatini S, Kurtzman NA: Metabolic Alkalosis. In general
   reference 6, p 691.

1-G. Respiratory Alkalosis

Central Causes
Voluntary hyperventilation
Anxiety, pain
Hypoxia
Fever
Salicylate toxicity
Head trauma
Brain tumor
Central nervous system infection
Cerebrovascular accident
Pregnancy
Recovery phase of metabolic acidosis

Cardiopulmonary Causes
Congestive heart failure
Pneumonia
Pulmonary embolism
Interstitial lung disease
Adult respiratory distress syndrome
Congestive heart failure
High altitude

Other
Hepatic insufficiency
Sepsis (especially gram-negative)
Drugs
   Progesterone, medroxyprogesterone
   Xanthines (e.g., aminophylline)
   Catecholamines (massive amounts)
   Nicotine
Mechanical ventilation
Heat exposure (e.g., heat stroke)

References
1. Cohen JJ, Kassirer JP: Acid-Base Metabolism. In general reference 6, p 181.
2. Kaehny WD: Pathogenesis and Management of Respiratory and Mixed Acid-Base Disorders. In general reference 16, p 187.

1-H. Hypernatremia

Pure Water Loss
Inability to obtain or swallow water (e.g., coma, dementia, infancy)
Impaired thirst drive (e.g., hypothalamic lesion)
Increased insensible loss

Excessive Sodium Intake
Iatrogenic sodium administration
  Sodium bicarbonate (cardiac arrest, treatment of lactic acidosis)
  Hypertonic saline (therapeutic abortion)
Accidental or deliberate ingestion of large quantities of sodium (e.g., substitution of salt for sugar in infant formula)
Seawater ingestion or drowning
Mineralocorticoid or glucocorticoid excess
  Primary aldosteronism
  Cushing's syndrome
  Ectopic adrenocorticotropic hormone production

Loss of Water in Excess of Sodium (Without Concomitant Water Intake)
Gastrointestinal loss (e.g., vomiting, diarrhea, intestinal fistula)
Renal loss
  Central diabetes insipidus
    Head trauma
    Posthypophysectomy
    Tumor
    Granulomatous disease (sarcoidosis, tuberculosis, Wegener's, syphilis, histiocytosis)
    Central nervous system infection
    Vascular lesion (cerebrovascular accident, aneurysm, sickle cell disease, Sheehan's syndrome)
    Congenital
  Impaired renal concentrating ability
    Osmotic diuresis
      Diabetic ketoacidosis
      Chronic renal failure, especially interstitial disease (e.g., polycystic disease, medullary cystic disease)
      Partial urinary tract obstruction, postobstructive diuresis
      Diuretic phase of acute renal failure
      Mannitol

> Tube feedings
> Infant formula (especially cow's milk)

Excessive diuretic use
Hypokalemia
Hypercalcemia
Decreased protein intake
Prolonged, excessive water intake
Sickle cell disease or trait
Multiple myeloma
Amyloidosis
Sarcoidosis
Sjögren's syndrome
Nephrogenic diabetes insipidus, congenital

Drugs
  Alcohol
  Lithium
  Demeclocycline
  Phenytoin
  Propoxyphene
  Sulfonylurea hypoglycemic agents
  Amphotericin B
  Methoxyflurane
  Colchicine
  Vinblastine

Skin loss (e.g., burns, sweating)
Peritoneal dialysis

Essential Hypernatremia (Reset Osmostat)

References
1. Ross EJ, Christie SBM: Hypernatremia. *Medicine* 48:441, 1969.
2. Berl T, Schrier RW: Disorders of Water Metabolism. In general reference 16, p 1.

1-I. Hyponatremia

***Factitious Hyponatremia (Normal
Serum Osmolality)***
Hyperglycemia
Hyperlipidemia
Hyperproteinemia
Hypertonic infusion of poorly reabsorbed solute (e.g., man-
　　nitol)

***States with Decreased Extracellular Fluid
Volume (Loss of Hypotonic Fluid Coupled with
Water Intake)***
Gastrointestinal loss (e.g., vomiting, diarrhea)
Third-space loss (e.g., burns, sweating, hemorrhagic pan-
　　creatitis)
Renal loss
　　Diuretic use
　　Renal salt-wasting (e.g., advanced chronic renal failure,
　　　　interstitial disease, renal tubular acidosis)
　　Osmotic diuresis
　　Mineralocorticoid deficiency

States with Increased Extracellular Fluid Volume
Congestive heart failure
Cirrhosis and ascites
Nephrotic syndrome
Renal failure, acute or chronic

***States with Normal or Slightly Increased
Extracellular Fluid Volume***
Syndrome of inappropriate antidiuretic hormone (SIADH)
　　Central nervous system disease
　　　　Tumor
　　　　Trauma
　　　　Infection (meningitis, encephalitis, abscess)
　　　　Cerebrovascular accident (thrombosis or hemorrhage)
　　　　Guillain-Barré syndrome
　　　　Delirium tremens
　　　　Multiple sclerosis
　　Pulmonary disease
　　　　Tumor
　　　　Pneumonia
　　　　Lung abscess
　　　　Tuberculosis
　　Carcinoma (especially lung, pancreas, duodenum)
　　Pain, stress (e.g., postoperative state)

  Acute psychosis
  Adrenal insufficiency
  Hypothyroidism
  Positive-pressure ventilation
  Porphyria
Drugs
  Antidiuretic hormone and analogues
  Nicotine
  Sulfonylurea compounds (especially chlorpropamide)
  Morphine
  Barbiturates
  Isoproterenol
  Nonsteroidal anti-inflammatory drugs
  Acetaminophen
  Clofibrate
  Carbamazepine
  Phenothiazines (thioridazine, fluphenazine)
  Amitriptyline
  Colchicine
  Vincristine
  Cyclophosphamide
Psychogenic polydipsia with massive water intake (> 20–
    25 L/day)
Beer drinking (excessive) associated with malnutrition
Essential (reset osmostat)

References

1. Berl T, Schrier RW: Disorders of Water Metabolism. In
   general reference 16, p 1.
2. Rossi NF, Schrier RW: Hyponatremic States. In general
   reference 6, p 461.

1-J. Hyperkalemia

Pseudohyperkalemia
Tourniquet use
Hemolysis (in vitro)
Leukocytosis, thrombocytosis

Intracellular-to-Extracellular K^+ Shift
Acidosis
Heavy exercise
Beta-blocking agents
Insulin deficiency
Digitalis intoxication
Hyperkalemic periodic paralysis

K^+ Load (Especially in Presence of Renal Insufficiency)
K^+ supplements
K^+-rich foods
K^+-containing salt substitute
Intravenous K^+
K^+-containing drugs (e.g., potassium penicillin)
Transfusion of aged blood
Hemolysis
Gastrointestinal bleeding
Cell destruction post-chemotherapy (especially with leukemia, lymphoma, myeloma)
Rhabdomyolysis or crush injury
Extensive tissue necrosis or catabolic state

Decreased K^+ Excretion
Renal failure (acute or chronic)
Drugs
    K^+-sparing diuretics (spironolactone, triamterene, amiloride)
    Beta-blocking agents
    Nonsteroidal anti-inflammatory drugs
    Converting enzyme inhibitors (e.g., captopril)
Aldosterone deficiency (e.g., adrenal insufficiency, selective hypoaldosteronism)
Selective defect in renal K^+ excretion
    Pseudohypoaldosteronism
    Lupus erythematosus
    Sickle cell disease
    Obstructive uropathy
    Renal transplantation
    Congenital

References
1. DeFronzo RA: Hyperkalemic States. In general reference 6, p 547.
2. Gabow PA, Peterson LN: Disorders of Potassium Metabolism. In general reference 16, p 207.

1-K. Hypokalemia

Extracellular-to-intracellular K⁺ shifts
  Alkalosis
  Increased plasma insulin (e.g., treatment phase of diabetic ketoacidosis)
  Beta-adrenergic agonists
  Hypokalemic periodic paralysis
Decreased intake
  Poor dietary intake
  Geophagia
Gastrointestinal loss
  Vomiting, nasogastric suction
  Diarrhea, laxative or enema abuse
  Malabsorption
  Ureterosigmoidostomy, ileal loop
  Enteric fistula
  Villous adenoma
Renal loss
  Diuretic therapy
  Primary aldosteronism
  Secondary aldosteronism
    Malignant hypertension
    Renal artery stenosis
    Congestive heart failure
    Cirrhosis and ascites
    Adrenocorticotropic hormone (ACTH) or glucocorticoid excess (Cushing's disease, Cushing's syndrome, ectopic ACTH production)
    Bartter's syndrome
    Renin-secreting tumor (e.g., renal hemangiopericytoma)
  Licorice ingestion
  Excessive use of chewing tobacco
  Renal tubular acidosis
  Diuresis during recovery from obstruction or acute renal failure
  Osmotic diuresis

Drugs and toxins
   Carbenicillin, penicillin (large doses)
   Amphotericin B
   L-Dopa
   Lithium
   Thallium
  Hypomagnesemia
  Acute leukemia
  Congenital adrenal hyperplasia
Sweat loss
  Heavy exercise
  Heat stroke
States of rapid cellular synthesis
  Intravenous hyperalimentation
  Recovery from megaloblastic anemia

References
1. Raymond KH, Kunan RT: Hypokalemic States. In general reference 6, p 519.
2. Gabow PA, Peterson LN: Disorders of Potassium Metabolism. In general reference 16, p 207.

1-L. Hypercalcemia

Hemoconcentration (increased serum albumin)*
Hyperparathyroidism
  Primary
    Parathyroid adenoma
    Parathyroid hyperplasia
    Parathyroid carcinoma
    Multiple endocrine adenomatosis
  Secondary (e.g., chronic renal failure)
  Ectopic
Malignancy
  Bony metastases
  Humoral factors (e.g., parathyroid hormone–like substances, osteoclast activating factor)
  Calcium-binding globulin (multiple myeloma)*
Thiazide diuretics
Immobilization (in association with rapid bone turnover states, e.g., adolescence or Paget's disease)
Milk-alkali syndrome

Vitamin D intoxication
Vitamin A intoxication
Granulomatous disease (especially sarcoidosis, tuberculosis)
Hypophosphatemia
Recovery from rhabdomyolysis-induced acute renal failure
Hyperthyroidism
Adrenal insufficiency
Acromegaly
Lithium administration
Familial hypocalciuric hypercalcemia
Idiopathic infantile hypercalcemia
Blue-diaper syndrome
Hypophosphatasia
Metaphyseal chondrodysplasia

References
1. Benabe JE, Martinez-Maldonado M: Disorders of Calcium Metabolism. In general reference 6, p 759.
2. Popovtzer MM, Knochel JP: Disorders of Calcium, Phosphorus, Vitamin D, and Parathyroid Hormone Activity. In general reference 16, p 251.

*Normal serum ionized calcium.

1-M. Hypocalcemia

Hypoalbuminemia*
Vitamin D deficiency states
  Sunlight deficiency
  Dietary deficiency
  Malabsorption (see 6-G)
    Postgastrectomy
    Sprue
    Pancreatic insufficiency
    Hepatobiliary disease with bile salt deficiency
    Laxative abuse
  Abnormal metabolism of vitamin D
    Renal failure (acute and chronic)
    Liver failure
    Vitamin D–dependent rickets
    Anticonvulsants, microsomal enzyme inducers

Hypoparathyroidism
  Congenital
  Idiopathic (infantile and adolescent-onset types)
  Acquired
    Surgical
    Iron overload (e.g., after multiple transfusions)
    Irradiation
    Neoplasm
Pseudohypoparathyroidism (types I and II)
Hyperphosphatemia
  Phosphate administration
    Enemas, laxatives
    Intravenous administration
    Cow's milk in infants
  Renal failure (chronic or acute)
  Rhabdomyolysis
  Cytotoxic therapy for leukemia, lymphoma
Malignancy
  Osteoblastic metastases (especially carcinoma of prostate, breast)
  Malignancy with increased thyrocalcitonin levels (especially medullary carcinoma of thyroid)
Magnesium depletion (see 1-Q)
Drugs
  Loop diuretics
  Agents causing decreased bone resorption (e.g., actinomycin, calcitonin, mithramycin)
  Calcium-complexing agents (e.g., citrate, EDTA)
Massive transfusion, plasma exchange
Acute pancreatitis
Healing phase of rickets, osteitis fibrosa, thyrotoxic osteopathy ("hungry bone syndrome")
Hyperkalemic periodic paralysis, acute
Osteopetrosis
Neonatal tetany

References

1. Benabe JE, Martinez-Maldonado M: Disorders of Calcium Metabolism. In general reference 6, p 759.
2. Popovtzer MM, Knochel JP: Disorders of Calcium, Phosphorus, Vitamin D, and Parathyroid Hormone Activity. In general reference 16, p 251.

*Normal serum ionized calcium.

1-N. Hyperphosphatemia

Decreased Excretion and/or Increased Load
Renal failure (acute or chronic)
Oral or intravenous phosphate
Phosphate-containing laxatives, enemas
Transfusion of stored blood
Acidosis (especially lactic acidosis or diabetic ketoacidosis)
Rhabdomyolysis
Cytotoxic therapy for malignancy
Hemolysis, resolving hematoma
Increased intestinal absorption (e.g., vitamin D intoxication)
Malignant hyperpyrexia
Phosphorus burns
Familial (rare)

Increased Renal Tubular Reabsorption
Hypoparathyroidism
Pseudohypoparathyroidism
Hyperthyroidism
Volume contraction
High atmospheric temperature
Postmenopausal state
Diphosphonate therapy
Acromegaly
Juvenile hypogonadism
Tumoral calcinosis

Reference
1. Brautbar N, Kleeman CR: Hypophosphatemia and Hyperphosphatemia: Clinical and Pathophysiologic Aspects. In general reference 6, p 789.

1-O. Hypophosphatemia

***Decreased Intake and Absorption and/or
Increased Nonrenal Loss***
Phosphate-binding antacids
Starvation, cachexia
Vomiting
Diarrhea, malabsorption
Hemodialysis

Transcellular Shift
Glucose infusion (with or without insulin administration)
Nutritional recovery syndrome
Alkalosis, respiratory
Androgens, anabolic steroids
Catecholamines (excessive secretion)
Infusion of:
   Bicarbonate
   Lactate
   Glucagon
Sepsis (especially gram-negative)
Thyrotoxicosis
Heat stroke
Gout, acute
Salicylate poisoning
Pregnancy
Myocardial infarction, acute

Renal Loss
Hyperparathyroidism, primary
Diuretic therapy
Volume expansion (including hyperaldosteronism)
Hypokalemia
Hypomagnesemia
Steroid therapy, Cushing's syndrome
Estrogens, oral contraceptives
Acidosis (especially metabolic)
Renal transplantation
Renal tubular defects (e.g., Fanconi syndrome, vitamin D–
   resistant rickets)
Tumor phosphaturia (mesenchymoma, neurofibroma, pleo-
   morphic sarcoma, sclerosing or cavernous hemangi-
   oma)

Multiple Mechanisms
Alcoholism and alcoholic withdrawal
Diabetic ketoacidosis

Liver disease, hepatic coma
Hyperalimentation
Vitamin D deficiency
Recovery from severe burns

References

1. Brautbar N, Kleeman CR: Hypophosphatemia and Hyperphosphatemia: Clinical and Pathophysiologic Aspects. In general reference 6, p 789.
2. Popovtzer MM, Knochel JP: Disorders of Calcium, Phosphorus, Vitamin D, and Parathyroid Hormone Activity. In general reference 16, p 251.

1-P. Hypermagnesemia

Renal failure, acute and chronic
Increased magnesium load (especially in presence of renal insufficiency)
  Magnesium-containing laxatives, antacids, or enemas
  Treatment of eclampsia (mother and infant)
  Diabetic ketoacidosis
Increased renal magnesium reabsorption
  Hyperparathyroidism
  Familial hypocalciuric hypercalcemia
  Hypothyroidism
  Mineralocorticoid deficiency, adrenal insufficiency

References

1. Brautbar N, Massry SG: Hypomagnesemia and Hypermagnesemia. In general reference 6, p 831.
2. Alfrey AC: Normal and Abnormal Magnesium Metabolism. In general reference 16, p 331.

1-Q. Hypomagnesemia

Redistribution
Postparathyroidectomy
Correction of metabolic acidosis (especially diabetic ketoacidosis)
Intravenous glucose, hyperalimentation
Refeeding after starvation
Acute pancreatitis

Decreased Intake and/or Increased Extrarenal Loss
Alcoholism
Malnutrition, poor intake
Nasogastric suction
Diarrhea, malabsorption (especially involving distal ileum)
Small bowel resection
Intestinal or biliary fistula
Profuse sweating, burns
Lactation

Increased Renal Loss
Drugs
  Diuretics
  Aminoglycosides
  Cisplatin
  Amphotericin B
Alcohol abuse
Diabetic ketoacidosis
Saline or osmotic diuresis
Postobstructive or post–acute renal failure diuresis
Tubulointerstitial renal disease
Hypercalcemic states
Primary or secondary aldosteronism
Potassium depletion
Hypoparathyroidism
Hyperthyroidism
Syndrome of inappropriate antidiuretic hormone secretion
Familial

References
1. Brautbar N, Massry SG: Hypomagnesemia & Hypermagnesemia. In general reference 6, p 831.
2. Alfrey AC: Normal and Abnormal Magnesium Metabolism. In general reference 16, p 331.

2 CARDIOVASCULAR SYSTEM

2-A. Chest Pain

Skin and subcutaneous lesions (including adiposis dolorosa, thrombophlebitis of thoracoepigastric vein [Mondor's disease])
Breast lesions
    Fibroadenosis
    Chronic cystic mastitis
    Acute breast abscess or mastitis
    Carcinoma
Musculoskeletal disorders
    Bruised or fractured rib
    Periostitis
    Periosteal hematoma
    Costochondritis (Tietze's syndrome)
    Slipping costal cartilage
    Intercostal muscle "stitch" or cramp
    Intercostal myositis
    Pectoral or other muscular strain
    Shoulder girdle disorders
    Cervical disk herniation
    Dorsal spine osteoarthritis
    Thoracic outlet syndromes

Neuralgia
  Herpes zoster
  Tabes dorsalis
  Neurofibroma
  Neoplasm
Pericardial disease
  Pericarditis (see 2-I)
  Neoplasm
  Congenital absence of left pericardium
Mediastinal disease
  Mediastinal emphysema
  Neoplasm
  Mediastinitis
Cardiovascular disease
  Acute myocardial infarction
  Angina pectoris
  Aortic valvular disease
  Idiopathic hypertrophic subaortic stenosis (IHSS)
  Mitral valve prolapse
  Acute aortic dissection
  Thoracic aortic aneurysm
  Myocarditis
  Primary pulmonary hypertension
  Ruptured sinus of Valsalva aneurysm
Pleural or pulmonary disease
  Pleuritis of any etiology (see 13-F)
  Tracheobronchitis
  Pneumonia
  Pulmonary thromboembolism
  Neoplasm
    Bronchogenic carcinoma
    Metastatic tumor
    Mesothelioma
  Other parenchymal lesions
Gastrointestinal disease
  Esophageal lesions
    Esophagitis
    Esophageal spasm
    Mallory-Weiss syndrome
    Esophageal rupture
    Foreign body
    Carcinoma
    Zenker's diverticulum
    Plummer-Vinson syndrome
  Peptic ulcer disease (with or without perforation)
  Biliary disease
    Acute cholecystitis
    Biliary colic

Pancreatitis
Subphrenic abscess
Splenic infarct
Thyroiditis
Psychogenic causes

References
1. General reference 4, p 227.
2. Braunwald E: Chest Discomfort and Palpitation. In general reference 1, p 17.

2-B. Edema

Localized
Venous or lymphatic obstruction
    Venous thrombosis
    Tumor invasion or compression (e.g., superior vena cava syndrome)
    Surgical or radiation damage
    Filariasis
Inflammatory disease
Allergic process
Physical or chemical trauma
Stings and bites
Immobilized or paralyzed limb
Congenital lymphedema

Generalized
Biventricular congestive heart failure
Cor pulmonale (see 13-O)
Pericardial disease
    Chronic constrictive pericarditis
    Pericardial effusion
Hypoalbuminemic states
    Hepatic cirrhosis
    Nephrotic syndrome
    Protein-losing enteropathy
    Malnutrition
    Severe chronic disease
Acute and chronic renal failure with volume overload
Inferior vena cava obstruction
Myxedema
Pregnancy
Iatrogenic salt overload
    Enteral feeding

Intravenous fluid administration
Drugs
    Carbenicillin and similar drugs
    Tamoxifen
    Corticosteroids
    Minoxidil
    Guanethidine
    Diazoxide
Trichinosis
Idiopathic cyclic edema
Hereditary angioneurotic edema

Reference
1. Braunwald E: Edema. In general reference 1, p 149.

2-C. Palpitation*

Palpitation Without Arrhythmia
Noncardiac disorders
  Anxiety
  Exercise
  Anemia
  Fever
  Volume depletion
  Thyrotoxicosis
  Menopausal syndrome
  Hypoglycemia
  Pheochromocytoma
  Aortic aneurysm
  Migraine syndrome
  Arteriovenous fistula
  Diaphragmatic flutter
  Drugs
    Sympathomimetic agents
    Ganglionic blockers
    Digitalis
    Nitrates
    Aminophylline
    Atropine
    Coffee, tea
    Tobacco
    Alcohol
    Thyroid extract
Cardiac disorders
  Aortic regurgitation

Aortic stenosis
Patent ductus arteriosus
Ventricular septal defect
Atrial septal defect
Marked cardiomegaly
Acute left ventricular failure
Hyperkinetic heart syndrome
Tricuspid insufficiency
Pericarditis
Prosthetic heart valve
Electronic pacemaker

Palpitation with Arrhythmia†
Extrasystoles
Bradyarrhythmias
Tachyarrhythmias

Reference
1. Braunwald E: Chest Discomfort and Palpitation. In general reference 1, p 17.

*Palpitation is the sensation of disturbed heartbeat. This entry was modified from Shander D: Palpitation and Disorders of Heartbeat. In Friedman HH (Ed): *Problem-Oriented Medical Diagnosis* (3rd ed.). Boston: Little, Brown, 1983, p 108.
†See 2-O.

2-D. Hypertension*

Systolic and Diastolic
Pseudohypertension (e.g., wrong-sized cuff)
Primary (essential)
Renal causes
   Parenchymal
   Vascular
   Renoprival (following bilateral nephrectomy)
   Renin-producing tumor
   Liddle's syndrome
Endocrine causes
   Acromegaly
   Hypothyroidism
   Hypercalcemia
   Adrenal causes
      Congenital adrenal hyperplasia
      Cushing's syndrome
      Primary aldosteronism
      Pheochromocytoma
   Extraadrenal chromaffin tumors
   Exogenous
      Oral contraceptives
      Estrogens
      Glucocorticoids
      Mineralocorticoids (e.g., licorice)
      Sympathomimetic agents
      Tyramine-containing foods and monoamine oxidase in-
         hibitors
Coarctation of aorta
Pregnancy-induced
Neurogenic causes
   Increased intracranial pressure
   Postoperative state
   Acute porphyria
   Lead poisoning
   Quadriplegia (acute)
   Diencephalic syndrome
   Familial dysautonomia
Increased intravascular volume
   Polycythemia vera
   Iatrogenic causes
Burns
Sleep apnea
Psychogenic causes
Drug withdrawal

Systolic
Increased cardiac output and/or stroke volume
   Aortic valvular regurgitation
   Fever
   Arteriovenous fistula, patent ductus arteriosus
   Paget's disease
   Beriberi
   Thyrotoxicosis (endogenous or exogenous)
   Anemia
   Hyperkinetic circulation
   Anxiety
   Complete heart block
Aortic rigidity

References
1. Kaplan NM: Systemic Hypertension: Mechanisms and Diagnosis. In general reference 7, p 819.
2. Williams GH, Braunwald E: Hypertensive Vascular Disease. In general reference 1, p 1024.

*Modified from Kaplan NM: Systemic Hypertension: Mechanisms and Diagnosis. In general reference 7, p 849.

2-E. Jugular Venous Distention

Extrathoracic Causes
Local venous obstruction of any cause (e.g., cervical goiter)
Circulatory overload of noncardiac etiology

Intrathoracic Causes
Valsalva maneuver
Retrosternal goiter
Superior vena cava syndrome
   Benign
   Malignant
Pericardial disease (see 2-I, 2-J)
   Cardiac tamponade
   Constrictive pericarditis
Cardiac disease
   Right heart failure of any etiology (see 2-G)
   Restrictive cardiomyopathy
   Right atrial myxoma
   Hyperkinetic heart circulatory states

Pleuropulmonary disease
  Pulmonary hypertension of any etiology (see 13-O)
  Bronchial asthma
  Chronic bronchitis and emphysema
  Tension pneumothorax

References
1. General reference 4, p 409.
2. Friedman HH: Venous Pressure. In general reference 3,
   p 40.

2-F. Heart Murmurs*

Systolic
Early systolic
  Physiologic (innocent)
  Small ventricular septal defect
  Large ventricular septal defect with pulmonary hyperten-
    sion
  Severe acute mitral or tricuspid regurgitation
  Tricuspid regurgitation without pulmonary hypertension
Midsystolic
  Physiologic (innocent)
    Vibratory murmur
    Pulmonary ejection murmur
    Aortic ejection murmur of old age
  Obstruction to left ventricular outflow
    Valvular aortic stenosis
    Fibrous subaortic stenosis
    Supravalvular aortic stenosis
    Idiopathic hypertrophic subaortic stenosis
    Aortic valve prosthesis
  Aortic dilatation
  Transmitted murmur of mitral regurgitation
  Aortic flow murmur in aortic regurgitation
  Coarctation of aorta
  Supraclavicular arterial bruit
  Obstruction to right ventricular outflow
    Pulmonic valvular stenosis
    Subpulmonic (infundibular) stenosis
  Flow murmur of atrial septal defect
  Idiopathic dilatation of pulmonary artery
  Pulmonary hypertension of any cause (occasionally)
Late systolic
  Mitral valve prolapse

Tricuspid valve prolapse
Holosystolic
  Mitral regurgitation
  Tricuspid regurgitation secondary to pulmonary hypertension
  Ventricular septal defect
  Patent ductus arteriosus with pulmonary hypertension

Diastolic
Early diastolic
  Aortic regurgitation
  Pulmonic regurgitation associated with pulmonary hypertension
Middiastolic
  Mitral stenosis
  Mitral valve prosthesis
  Tricuspid stenosis
  Atrial myxoma
  Left atrial ball-valve thrombus
  Austin Flint murmur
  Increased diastolic atrioventricular flow
    Mitral and tricuspid regurgitation
    Left-to-right shunt (e.g., ventricular septal defect)
    Acute rheumatic valvulitis
  Coronary artery stenosis
Presystolic
  Mitral stenosis
  Tricuspid stenosis
  Atrial myxoma
  Left-to-right shunt
  Complete heart block
  Severe pulmonic stenosis
  Fourth heart sound

Continuous
Pseudomurmur (e.g., pericardial friction rub)
Traumatic or surgical arteriovenous fistula
Patent ductus arteriosus
Surgically created aorticopulmonary fistula
Pulmonary arteriovenous fistula
Aorticopulmonary window without severe pulmonary hypertension
Pulmonary embolism
Coronary arteriovenous fistula
Ruptured sinus of Valsalva aneurysm
Coarctation of aorta
Bronchial artery collateral circulation
Lutembacher's syndrome

Cervical venous hum
Mammary souffle
Aortic arch syndrome
Pulmonary artery branch stenosis

References
1. Craige E: Echophonocardiography and Other Noninvasive Techniques to Elucidate Heart Murmurs. In general reference 7, p 65.
2. O'Rourke RA, Braunwald E: Physical Examination of the Heart. In general reference 1, p 865.
3. Friedman HH: Cardiovascular Problems: Heart Murmurs. In general reference 3, p 66.

*See also 2-N.

2-G. Congestive Heart Failure

Left Heart Failure
Hypertensive heart disease
Coronary artery disease
Acute myocardial infarction
Aortic and mitral valvular disease
Cardiomyopathy (see 2-H)
Arrhythmias
Congenital heart disease
Endocarditis
Cardiotoxic drugs (e.g., Adriamycin)
Myocarditis
Acute rheumatic fever
Traumatic heart disease
Thyrotoxicosis
Thiamine deficiency
Anemia
Arteriovenous fistula (e.g., Paget's disease)
Neoplastic heart disease
Toxic shock syndrome
Pulmonary thromboembolism
Postcardioversion

Right Heart Failure (see 13-O)
Associated with pulmonary venous hypertension (postcapillary)
  Cardiac disease (see above)

Pulmonary venous disease
  Mediastinal neoplasm or granuloma
  Mediastinitis
  Anomalous pulmonary venous return
  Congenital pulmonary venous stenosis
  Idiopathic pulmonary veno-occlusive disease
Associated with pulmonary arterial hypertension (precapillary)
  Lung and pleural disease
    Chronic bronchitis, emphysema, and asthma
    Granulomatous disease (e.g., sarcoidosis)
    Fibrotic disease
    Neoplasm
    Chronic suppurative disease (e.g., bronchiectasis)
    Collagen-vascular disease
    Other restrictive processes (see 13-N)
    Following lung resection
    Fibrothorax
    Chest wall deformity
      Kyphoscoliosis
      Thoracoplasty
  Alveolar hypoventilation
    Neuromuscular
    Primary alveolar hypoventilation
    Obesity
    Sleep apnea syndrome
    High-altitude pulmonary hypertension
  Intracardiac disease
    Increased flow associated with large left-to-right shunt
      Patent ductus arteriosus
      Atrial septal defect
      Ventricular septal defect
      Sinus of Valsalva aneurysm
    Decreased flow
      Tetralogy of Fallot
      Peripheral pulmonary artery stenosis (or stenoses)
      Unilateral absence or stenosis of pulmonary artery
  Vascular disease
    Pulmonary thromboembolic disease
      Thrombotic
      Septic
      Fat
      Air
      Amniotic fluid, trophoblastic
      Foreign material (e.g., talc)
      Parasitic
      Metastatic neoplasm

Thrombosis associated with SS and SC hemoglobin
Thrombosis associated with eclampsia
Primary pulmonary hypertension
Pulmonary arteritis
Raynaud's disease
Scleroderma
CRST syndrome
Schistosomiasis
Rheumatoid arthritis
Systemic lupus erythematosus
Polymyositis, dermatomyositis
Granulomatous arteritis (e.g., Wegener's)
Takayasu's disease
Without pulmonary hypertension
Pulmonic stenosis
Tricuspid stenosis (nonrheumatic)
Tricuspid regurgitation not associated with pulmonary hypertension
Decreased right ventricular compliance
Ebstein's anomaly
Atrial myxoma

References
1. General reference 24, p 1203.
2. Moser KM (Ed): *Pulmonary Vascular Diseases.* New York: Marcel Dekker, 1979.
3. Grossman W, Braunwald E: Pulmonary Hypertension. In general reference 7, p 793.

2-H. Cardiomyopathy

Congestive
Congenital
   Diabetes
   Familial
   Duchenne's muscular dystrophy
   Facioscapulohumeral muscular dystrophy
   Limb-girdle muscular dystrophy
   Myotonic dystrophy
   Refsum's disease
   Glycogen storage disorders
   Mucopolysaccharidoses
   Fabry's disease
   Gaucher's disease
Acquired
   Idiopathic
   Alcoholism
   Myocarditis
   Peripartum
   Acquired immunodeficiency syndrome (AIDS)
   Uremia
   Obesity
   Sarcoidosis
   Hyperthermia
   Hypothermia
   Transplant rejection
   Irradiation
   Acromegaly
   Hypophosphatemia
   Hypocalcemia
   Hemochromatosis
   Polymyositis, dermatomyositis
   Vasculitis (e.g., Wegener's granulomatosis)
   Whipple's disease
   Amyloidosis
   Scleroderma
   Hypoxia
   Neoplasm
   Becker's disease
   Nutritional deficiency (e.g., thiamine, selenium)
   Endomyocardial fibrosis
   Toxins, drugs
      Disopyramide
      Daunorubicin
      Doxorubicin (Adriamycin)
      Cyclophosphamide

5-Fluorouracil
Phosphate (poisoning)
Phenothiazines
Lithium
Carbon monoxide
Emetine
Miconazole
Chloroquine
Acetaminophen, paracetamol
Lead
Arsenic
Hydrocarbons
Antimony
Cobalt
Snake or insect bites

Restrictive
Pseudocardiomyopathy (i.e., constrictive pericarditis)
Amyloidosis
Hemochromatosis
Sarcoidosis
Scleroderma
Neoplasm
Endocardial fibroelastosis
Loeffler's fibroplastic endocarditis (hypereosinophilic syndrome)
Endomyocardial fibrosis

Hypertrophic
Idiopathic hypertrophic subaortic stenosis (IHSS)
Glycogen storage disease (Pompe's disease)
Friedreich's ataxia
Lentiginosis

References
1. Wynne J, Braunwald E: The Cardiomyopathies and Myocarditides. In general reference 7, p 1410.
2. Goodwin JF: Congestive and Hypertrophic Cardiomyopathies: A Decade of Study. *Lancet* 1:731, 1970.

2-I. Pericarditis*

Idiopathic†
Infection
  Viral†
  Bacterial†
  Mycobacterial†
  Mycoplasmal
  Fungal†
  Parasitic†
  Spirochetal (e.g., Lyme disease)
Acute myocardial infarction
Uremia†
Neoplasm†
Aortic dissection with hemopericardium
Connective-tissue or hypersensitivity diseases†
  Post–myocardial infarction (Dressler's syndrome)
  Postpericardiectomy
  Drugs
    Penicillin
    Isoniazid
    Methysergide
    Daunorubicin
    Emetine
    Cromolyn
    Minoxidil
    Bleomycin
    Cyclosphosphamide
  Systemic lupus erythematosus
    Idiopathic
    Drug-related (e.g., hydralazine, procainamide)
  Mixed connective-tissue disease
  Scleroderma
  Wegener's granulomatosis
  Rheumatoid arthritis
  Polyarteritis nodosa
  Polymyositis
  Reiter's syndrome
  Serum sickness
  Acute rheumatic fever
Trauma†
  Penetrating wounds
  Catheter- or pacemaker-induced cardiac perforation
  Blunt chest trauma
  Cardiopulmonary resuscitation
  Cardiothoracic surgery
  Cardioversion

Pseudoaneurysm Neptune
Cholesterol pericarditis
   Idiopathic
   Rheumatoid arthritis
   Hypercholesterolemia
   Myxedema
   Tuberculosis
Talc or other foreign substance
Sarcoidosis
Postirradiation†
Esophageal rupture
Uncommon miscellaneous etiologies
   Congenital heart disease (e.g., atrial septal defect)
   Familial Mediterranean fever
   Right atrial myxoma
   Degos' disease
   Gaucher's disease
   Myeloid metaplasia
   Silicosis
   Scorpion fish sting
   Pseudomyxoma peritonei
   Severe chronic anemia (e.g., thalassemia)
   Pancreatitis
   Whipple's disease
   Acute gouty arthritis
   Pulmonary thromboembolism
   Takayasu's disease
   Mulibrey nanism†
   Nontraumatic hemopericardium

References
1. Lorell BH, Braunwald E: Pericardial Disease. In general
   reference 7, p 1484.
2. Braunwald E: Pericardial Disease. In general reference
   1, p 1008.

*See also 2-J.
†May be commonly associated with development of constrictive pericarditis.

2-J. Pericardial Effusion

Pericarditis (see 2-I)
Congestive heart failure
Hypoalbuminemia
Acute pancreatitis
Chylopericardium*
Hemopericardium†
Myxedema*

References
1. Lorell BH, Braunwald E: Pericardial Disease. In general
   reference 7, p 1484.
2. Roberts WC, Spray TL: Pericardial Heart Disease. *Curr
   Prob Cardiol* 2(3):55, 1977.

*May be associated with chronic constrictive pericarditis.
†May be associated with acute cardiac tamponade.

2-K. Hypotension and Shock

Hypovolemia
  External losses
    Hemorrhage
    Gastrointestinal loss
    Renal loss
      Diuretics
      Diabetes insipidus
      Osmotic diuresis (e.g., diabetes mellitus)
      Diuretic phase of acute renal failure
      Salt-losing nephropathy
      Postobstructive diuresis
    Cutaneous loss
      Burns
      Exudative lesions
      Perspiration and insensible loss without replacement
  Internal losses
    Hemorrhage (e.g., anticoagulant therapy)
      Hemothorax
      Hemoperitoneum
      Retroperitoneal hemorrhage
      Fracture
    Fluid sequestration
      Ascites

      Bowel obstruction
      Peritonitis
      Phlegmon (e.g., pancreatitis)
Cardiovascular causes
  Arrhythmia (see 2-O)
  Regurgitant lesions
    Acute mitral or aortic regurgitation
    Rupture of interventricular septum
    Giant left ventricular aneurysm
  Obstructive lesions
    Valvular stenosis
    Hypertrophic cardiomyopathy
    Atrial myxoma
    Intracardiac or valvular thrombus
  Myopathy
    Acute myocardial infarction
    Dilated or restrictive cardiomyopathy
    Other myocardial disorders (associated with low cardiac output)
  Pericardial disease
    Cardiac tamponade
    Constrictive pericarditis
  Aortic lesions
    Acute dissection
    Coarctation
    Rupture (e.g., trauma or aneurysm)
  Vena cava obstruction
Pleuropulmonary disease
  Tension pneumothorax
  Pulmonary embolism (including thrombus, amniotic fluid, air, tumor)
  Primary or secondary pulmonary hypertension
  Eisenmenger reaction
Infection
  Septicemia
  Specific infections (e.g., dengue fever)
  Toxic shock syndrome
Anaphylaxis
Endocrine disease
  Adrenal insufficiency
  Hypoglycemia or hyperglycemia
  Hypocalcemia or hypercalcemia
  Myxedema or thyroid storm
  Pheochromocytoma
  Pituitary failure including diabetes insipidus
Hypoxia
Severe acidosis or alkalosis
Nonbacterial sepsis syndrome

Hypothermia or hyperthermia
Hepatic failure
Drugs and toxins
   Drug overdose and poisoning (e.g., barbiturates)
   Antihypertensive agents
   Other vasodilators (e.g., nitroglycerin)
   Heavy metals
Hyperviscosity syndrome
Neuropathic causes
   Brainstem failure
   Spinal cord dysfunction
   Autonomic insufficiency

References
1. Dole WP, O'Rourke RA: Hypotension and Cardiogenic Shock. In Stein JH (Ed): *Internal Medicine* (2nd ed). Boston: Little, Brown, 1983, p 407.
2. Weil MH, Planta MV, Rackow EC: Acute Circulatory Failure (Shock). In general reference 7, p 561.

2-L. Cardiac Arrest (Sudden Cardiopulmonary Collapse)

Arrhythmia (with or without digitalis intoxication)
   Tachyarrhythmia
      Ventricular fibrillation (e.g., prolonged QT syndromes)
      Ventricular tachycardia
   Bradyarrhythmia
      Sinus bradycardia
      Junctional rhythm
      Atrioventricular block
      Idioventricular rhythm
   Asystole
Upper airway obstruction
   Structural lesion
   Sleep apnea syndromes
   Foreign body
Acute respiratory failure with hypoxemia and/or hypercarbia
Hypoxia of any cause (e.g., carbon monoxide poisoning)
Pulmonary hypertension
Severe acidosis or alkalosis
Hypoglycemia
Syncope (see 12-D)
Addisonian crisis

Drug overdose, allergy, or adverse reaction
  Narcotics
  Insulin
  Sedatives
  Quinidine
  Disopyramide
  Procainamide and other antiarrhythmics
  Phenothiazines
  Tricyclic antidepressants
  Nitrates
  Aminophylline
  Propranolol
  Warfarin
  Penicillins
  Sulfonamides
  Antihypertensive agents
Shock of any etiology (see also 2-K), especially:
  Hypovolemia
  Tension pneumothorax
  Cardiac tamponade or pericardial constriction
  Anaphylaxis
  Sepsis
  Aortic dissection or rupture
  Pulmonary embolism (of any type)
  Acute myocardial infarction
  Other common cardiac causes
    Severe coronary heart disease
    Valvular disease (e.g., aortic stenosis)
    Myocarditis and cardiomyopathy
    Cardiac rupture
    Mitral valve prolapse
    Primary conduction system or nodal disease
Electrolyte abnormality (especially potassium, calcium,
    magnesium)
Hypothermia or hyperthermia
Electric shock
Insect stings and bites
Neurologic disorders
  Stroke
  Seizure
  Brainstem compression of any cause
  Infection
Sudden infant death syndrome
Liquid protein diet
Modified fast diet programs

References
1. Myerburg RJ, Castellanos A: Cardiovascular Arrest and

Sudden Cardiac Death. In general reference 7, p 742.
2. Sobel BE, Braunwald E: Sudden Cardiovascular Collapse and Death. In general reference 1, **p 158.**

2-M. Complications of Cardiopulmonary Resuscitation

Cerebral
  Hypoxic encephalopathy
Oronasopharyngeal
  Laceration
  Fractured teeth
  Epistaxis
Neck
  Spinal cord injury
  Vascular injury and hematoma
Lung and chest wall
  Pneumothorax and pneumomediastinum
  Subcutaneous emphysema
  Rib and sternal fractures
  Hemothorax
  Atelectasis
    Malpositioned endotracheal tube
    Foreign body
    Secretions
  Aspiration
Heart and pericardium
  Hemopericardium and cardiac tamponade
  Lacerated heart or coronary vessels
  Ruptured ventricle
Visceral injury
  Acute gastric dilatation
  Gastroesophageal, liver, or splenic laceration
Acute renal failure
Fat embolism
Volume overload
Metabolic alkalosis
  Sodium bicarbonate administration
  Posthypercapnic
Bacteremia

Reference
1. Myerburg RJ, Castellanos A: Cardiovascular Arrest and Sudden Cardiac Death. In general reference 7, p 742.

2-N. Valvular Disease*

Aortic Valve
Stenosis
  Valvular
    Congenital
    Rheumatic
    Calcific (senile)
    Atherosclerotic
    Rheumatoid
    Ochronosis
  Supravalvular
  Subvalvular
Regurgitation
  Congenital
    Bicuspid aortic valve
     Isolated
     Associated with:
      Coarctation
      Ventricular septal defect
      Patent ductus arteriosus
    Tricuspid aortic valve
     Isolated
     Associated with:
      Ventricular septal defect
      Valvular aortic stenosis
      Supravalvular aortic stenosis
      Subvalvular aortic stenosis
      Congenital aneurysm of sinus of Valsalva
      Cusp fenestrations
    Quadricuspid aortic valve
  Acquired
    Valvular
     Rheumatic heart disease
     Bacterial endocarditis
     Calcific aortic valve disease
     Atherosclerosis
     Traumatic valve rupture
     Postaortic valve surgery
      Postvalvulotomy
      Leakage around prosthesis
      Endocarditis
     Miscellaneous
      Ankylosing spondylitis
      Reiter's syndrome
      Rheumatoid arthritis

Systemic lupus erythematosus
Scleroderma
Myxomatous degeneration
Pseudoxanthoma elasticum
Mucopolysaccharidoses
Osteogenesis imperfecta
Cusp fenestrations
Methysergide
Aortic dilatation or distortion
Senile dilatation
Cystic medial necrosis with or without Marfan's syndrome
Takayasu's disease
Relapsing polychondritis
Syphilis
Ankylosing spondylitis
Psoriatic arthritis
Ulcerative colitis with arthritis
Reiter's syndrome
Giant-cell arteritis
Ehlers-Danlos syndrome
Hypertension
Cogan's syndrome

Mitral Valve
Stenosis
Congenital
Rheumatic
Carcinoid syndrome
Marantic endocarditis
Systemic lupus erythematosus
Calcific
Lutembacher's syndrome
Rheumatoid arthritis
Hunter-Hurler disease
Methysergide
Regurgitation
Congenital
Isolated mitral regurgitation
Idiopathic hypertrophic subaortic stenosis (IHSS)
Connective-tissue disorders
Ehlers-Danlos syndrome
Hurler's syndrome
Marfan's syndrome
Pseudoxanthoma elasticum
Osteogenesis imperfecta

Atrioventricular cushion defect
Endocardial fibroelastosis
Parachute mitral valve complex
Hypoplastic left heart syndrome
Anomalous left coronary artery from pulmonary artery
Congenital mitral stenosis
Corrected transposition of great vessels with or without
    Ebstein's malformation
Supravalvular ring of left atrium
Acquired
  Rheumatic
  Mitral valve prolapse syndrome
  Papillary muscle dysfunction (e.g., following myocar-
    dial infarction)
  Ruptured or abnormal chordae tendineae (e.g., idio-
    pathic)
  Bacterial endocarditis
  Calcified mitral annulus
  Left ventricular dilatation or aneurysm
  Aortic valve disease
  Prosthetic valve disruption
  Trauma
  Post–cardiac surgery
  Rheumatoid arthritis
  Ankylosing spondylitis
  Systemic lupus erythematosus
  Left atrial myxoma
  Spontaneous rupture
  Carcinoid syndrome
  Giant left atrium

Pulmonic Valve
Stenosis
  Congenital
    Valvular stenosis
    Valvular dysplasia (e.g., Noonan's syndrome)
    Tetralogy of Fallot
    Supravalvular aortic stenosis syndrome
  Acquired
    Intrinsic valvular lesions
      Rheumatic disease
      Carcinoid syndrome
      Endocarditis
      Primary neoplasm
    Extrinsic lesions
      Neoplasm
      Aortic or septal aneurysm

        Sinus of Valsalva aneurysm
        Constrictive pericarditis
Regurgitation
  Congenital
    Absent pulmonic valve
    Isolated pulmonic regurgitation
    Associated with:
      Tetralogy of Fallot
      Ventricular septal defect
      Pulmonic valvular stenosis
      Idiopathic dilatation of pulmonic valve
  Acquired
    Valve ring dilatation secondary to pulmonary hyperten-
        sion of any cause (see 2-G, Right Heart Failure)
    Pulmonary artery dilatation, idiopathic
    Bacterial endocarditis
    Post–pulmonic valve surgery
    Rheumatic disease
    Trauma
    Syphilis
    Carcinoid syndrome
    Marfan's syndrome

Tricuspid Valve
Stenosis
  Rheumatic heart disease
  Carcinoid syndrome
  Fibroelastosis
  Endomyocardial fibrosis
Regurgitation
  Right ventricular dilatation of any cause (e.g., mitral ste-
    nosis)
  Pulmonary hypertension (see 2-G, under Right Heart
    Failure)
  Rheumatic heart disease
  Right ventricular papillary muscle dysfunction
  Myxomatous valve and chordae (usually in association
    with mitral valve prolapse with or without atrial septal
    defect)
  Trauma
  Bacterial endocarditis
  Carcinoid syndrome
  Ebstein's anomaly
  Common atrioventricular canal
  Ventricular septal aneurysm
  Right atrial myxoma
  Constrictive pericarditis

Thyrotoxicosis
Isolated lesion
Following surgical excision
Marfan's syndrome

References
1. Braunwald E: Valvular Heart Disease. In general reference 7, p 1023.
2. Braunwald E: Valvular Heart Disease. In general reference 1, p 956.

*See also 2-F.

2-O. Arrhythmias

Premature Beats*
Extrasystole
  Sinus (rare)
  Atrial
  Atrioventricular junctional
  Ventricular
Parasystole
Capture beat
Reciprocal beat
Better atrioventricular conduction (e.g., 3 : 2), interrupting
    poorer (e.g., 2 : 1)
Supernormal conduction during advanced atrioventricular
    block
Rhythm resumption after inapparent bigeminy

Bradycardia (< 60 beats/min)†
Sinus bradycardia
Sinus arrhythmia
Wandering atrial pacemaker
Sinoatrial block (second and third degree)
Sinus pause or arrest
Nonconducted atrial bigeminy
Hypersensitive carotid sinus syndrome
Atrioventricular block (second and third degree)
Supraventricular tachyarrhythmias with high-grade atrio-
    ventricular block (rare)
Escape rhythms (resulting from bradycardia of any cause)
  Atrioventricular junctional
  Idioventricular
Sick sinus syndrome

Tachycardia (Ventricular Rate > 100 Beats/Min)

	Rate		Carotid sinus massage
	Atrial	Ventricular	
NORMAL QRS (< 0.10 SEC)			
Regular Rhythm			
Sinus tachycardia	100–200 (usually < 160)	100–200 (usually < 160)	Gradual slowing with return to previous rate
Paroxysmal supraventricular tachycardia[a]	140–250	140–250	No effect or abrupt termination
Paroxysmal atrial tachycardia with block	140–250	Variable (usually < 170)	May abruptly and transiently decrease ventricular rate; generally contraindicated
Atrial flutter	250–350	Variable (usually 120–175)	Transient slowing of ventricular rate, revealing flutter waves
Paroxysmal atrioventricular junctional tachycardia	140–250	140–250	No effect or abrupt termination
Nonparoxysmal atrioventricular junctional tachycardia	Depends on atrial mechanism	65–130	No effect or gradual slowing with return to previous rate; generally contraindicated

Tachycardia (Ventricular Rate > 100 Beats/Min) (continued)

	Rate		Carotid sinus massage
	Atrial	Ventricular	
NORMAL QRS (< 0.10 SEC)			
Irregular Rhythm			
Atrial fibrillation[a]	350–600	Variable	Transient decrease in ventricular rate
Paroxysmal atrial tachy-cardia with variable block	140–250	Variable	May abruptly and transiently de-crease ventricular rate; gener-ally contraindicated
Atrial flutter with variable block	250–350	Variable	Transient slowing of ventricular rate, revealing flutter waves
Multifocal atrial tachy-cardia	100–200	100–200	No effect or gradual slowing
ABNORMAL QRS (> 0.10 SEC)			
Regular Rhythm			
Sinus tachycardia with preexisting bundle-	100–200 (usually < 160)	100–200 (usually < 160)	Gradual slowing with return to previous rate

branch block or preexcitation			
Paroxysmal supraventricular tachycardia with aberrant conduction, preexisting bundle-branch block, or preexcitation (rare)	140–250	140–250	No effect or abrupt termination
Paroxysmal supraventricular tachycardia with block, with aberrant conduction or preexisting bundle-branch block	140–250	Variable (usually < 170)	May abruptly and transiently decrease ventricular rate; generally contraindicated
Atrial flutter with aberrant conduction or preexisting bundle-branch block	250–350	Variable (usually 120–175)	Transient slowing of ventricular rate, revealing flutter waves
Atrioventricular junctional tachycardias with aberrant conduction or preexisting bundle-branch block			

Tachycardia (Ventricular Rate > 100 Beats/Min) (continued)

	Rate		Carotid sinus massage
	Atrial	Ventricular	
ABNORMAL QRS (> 0.10 SEC)			
Regular Rhythm			
Paroxysmal	140–250	140–250	No effect or abrupt termination
Nonparoxysmal	Depends on atrial mechanism	65–130	No effect or gradual slowing with return to previous rate; generally contraindicated
Ventricular tachycardia	Equal to or less than ventricular rate	60–250 (usually > 150 and may be slightly irregular)	Atrial rate may slow; no effect on ventricular rate
Irregular Rhythm			
Atrial fibrillation with aberrant conduction or preexisting bundle-branch block	350–600	Variable	Transient decrease in ventricular rate
Paroxysmal supraventricular tachycardia with variable block,	140–250	Variable	May abruptly and transiently decrease ventricular rate; generally contraindicated

with aberrant conduction, or preexisting bundle-branch block		
Atrial flutter with variable block, with aberrant conduction or preexisting bundle-branch block	250–350	Variable	Transient slowing of ventricular rate, revealing flutter waves

[a]Arrhythmias most commonly associated with preexcitation (Wolff-Parkinson-White syndrome).

References

1. Marriott HJL: *Practical Electrocardiography* (6th ed). Baltimore, Md.: Williams & Wilkins, 1977.
2. Friedman HH: *Diagnostic Electrocardiography and Vectorcardiography* (2nd ed). New York: McGraw-Hill, 1977.
3. Zipes, DP: Specific Arrhythmias: Diagnosis and Treatment. In general reference 7, p 658.

2-P. Electrocardiographic Abnormalities

QRS Interval, Prolonged
Bundle-branch blocks
Nonspecific intraventricular conduction delay
Aberrant ventricular conduction
Ectopic ventricular rhythm (e.g., ventricular parasystole)
Drug effect (e.g., quinidine or procainamide)
Electrolyte abnormalities (hyperkalemia, hypokalemia, hypercalcemia, hypomagnesemia)
Preexcitation (Wolff-Parkinson-White syndrome)
Left ventricular enlargement
Periinfarction block
Hypothermia

ST Segment Changes
Elevation
  Normal variant (e.g., "early repolarization")
  Artifact
  Myocardial infarction
  Prinzmetal's angina
  Ventricular aneurysm
  Reciprocal changes
  Pericarditis
  Hyperkalemia (rarely)
  Bundle-branch block
  Acute cor pulmonale (e.g., pulmonary thromboembolism)
  Myocarditis
  Neoplastic heart disease
  Stroke
  Hypertrophic cardiomyopathy
  Hypothermia
Depression
  Nonspecific abnormality (e.g., anxiety, shock)
  Drugs
    Digitalis
    Tricyclic antidepressants
    Lithium
  Bundle-branch block
  Left or right ventricular strain
  Electrolyte abnormalities (hyperkalemia or hypokalemia)
  Subendocardial ischemia or infarction
  Mitral valve prolapse
  Tachycardia
  Myocarditis or cardiomyopathy
  Reciprocal changes
  Cerebral or subarachnoid injury

Pancreatitis or other acute intraabdominal catastrophe
Pulmonary thromboembolism
Hypothyroidism

QT Interval
Prolonged
    Electrolyte abnormalities (hypocalcemia, hypokalemia,
       ["QU" prolongation])
    Complete heart block
    Mitral valve prolapse
    Left ventricular enlargement
    Myocardial infarction and ischemia
    Myocarditis and cardiomyopathy
    Diffuse myocardial disease
    Cerebral or subarachnoid injury
    Drugs (e.g., quinidine, procainamide, phenothiazines)
    Hypothermia
    Heritable anomaly
    Alkalosis
Shortened
    Electrolyte abnormalities (hypercalcemia, hyperkalemia)
    Digitalis
    Acidosis

T-Wave Changes
Peaking
    Normal variant
    Nonspecific abnormality
    Electrolyte abnormalities (hyperkalemia, hypocalcemia,
       hypomagnesemia)
    Acute myocardial ischemia or infarction
    Reciprocal effect in strictly posterior myocardial infarction
    Left ventricular enlargement
    Anemia
Inversion
    Normal
    Juvenile T-wave pattern
    Left bundle-branch block
    Nonspecific abnormality
    Myocardial ischemia or infarction
    Myocarditis
    Pericarditis
    Ventricular strain
    Acute or chronic cor pulmonale
    Cerebral or subarachnoid injury
    Drugs (e.g., quinidine, phenothiazines)
    Electrolyte abnormalities (hypokalemia, hypocalcemia,
       hypomagnesemia)

Complete atrioventricular block
Vagotomy
Following tachycardia

Q Waves, Abnormal
Myocardial infarction
Dextrocardia or dextroversion
Reversal of right and left arm leads (lead I)
Ventricular enlargement
Acute and chronic cor pulmonale (e.g., pulmonary embolism)
Preexcitation
Cardiac surgery
Spontaneous pneumothorax (especially left)
Cardiomyopathy and myocarditis (e.g., hypertrophic cardiomyopathy)
Localized destructive myocardial disease (e.g., neoplasm)
Left bundle-branch block
Normal variant (rare)
Tachycardia (transitory)
Critical illness (e.g., pancreatitis)

References
1. Friedman HH: *Diagnostic Electrocardiography and Vectorcardiography* (2nd ed). New York: McGraw-Hill, 1977.
2. Marriott HJL: *Practical Electrocardiography* (6th ed). Baltimore, Md.: Williams & Wilkins, 1977.
3. Fisch C: Electrocardiography and Vectorcardiography. In general reference 7, p 180.

2-Q. Cardiac Risk Index for Noncardiac Surgical Procedures

Computation of the Cardiac Risk Index

Criteria	"Points"
1. History	
a. Age > 70 yr	**5**
b. MI in previous 6 mo	**10**
2. Physical examination	
a. S_3 gallop or JVD	**11**
b. Important VAS	**3**
3. Electrocardiogram	
a. Rhythm other than sinus or PACs on last preoperative ECG	**7**
b. > 5 PVCs/min documented at any time before operation	**7**
4. General status: PO_2 < 60 or PCO_2 > 50 mmHg, K < 3.0 or HCO_3 < 20 mEq/L, BUN > 50 or Cr > 3.0 mg/dl, abnormal SGOT, signs of chronic liver disease, or patient bedridden from noncardiac causes	**3**
5. Operation	
a. Intraperitoneal, intrathoracic, or aortic	**3**
b. Emergency	**4**
Total possible:	**53**

Key: MI = myocardial infarction; JVD = jugular vein distention; VAS = valvular aortic stenosis; PACs = premature atrial contractions; ECG = electrocardiogram; PVCs = premature ventricular contractions; PO_2 = partial pressure of oxygen; PCO_2 = partial pressure of carbon dioxide; K = potassium; HCO_3 = bicarbonate; BUN = blood urea nitrogen; Cr = creatinine; and SGOT = serum glutamic oxaloacetic transaminase.
Source: Adapted from Goldman L, Caldera DL, Nussbaum SR, et al: Multifactorial Index of Cardiac Risk in Non-cardiac Surgical Procedures. *N Engl J Med* 297:848, 1977. By permission of the *New England Journal of Medicine*.

Cardiac Risk Index

Class	Point total	No (or only minor) complications ($N = 943$)	Life-threatening complication[a] ($N = 39$)	Cardiac deaths ($N = 19$)
I ($N = 537$)	0–5	532 (99)[b]	4 (0.7)	1 (0.2)
II ($N = 316$)	6–12	295 (93)	16 (5)	5 (2)
III ($N = 130$)	13–25	112 (86)	15 (11)	3 (2)
IV ($N = 18$)	> 26	4 (22)	4 (22)	10 (56)

[a]Documented intraoperative or postoperative myocardial infarction, pulmonary edema, or ventricular tachycardia without progression to cardiac death.
[b]Figures in parentheses denote percentages.
Source: Goldman L, Caldera DL, Nussbaum SR, et al: Multifactorial Index of Cardiac Risk in Non-cardiac Surgical Procedures. *N Engl J Med* 297:848, 1977. Reprinted by permission of the *New England Journal of Medicine.*

References

1. Goldman L, Wolf MA, Braunwald E: General Anesthesia and Noncardiac Surgery in Patients with Heart Disease. In general reference 7, p. 1693.
2. Goldman L, Caldera DL, Nussbaum SR, et al: Multifactorial Index of Cardiac Risk in Non-cardiac Surgical Procedures. *N Engl J Med* 297:845, 1977.
3. Goldman L: Cardiac risks and complications of noncardiac surgery. *Ann Intern Med* 98:504, 1983.

3 DRUGS

3-A. Bacterial Endocarditis Prophylaxis in Adults

Antimicrobial regimens

A. Penicillin V, 2 gm PO 1 hr before procedure and 1 gm PO 6 hr after
B. Aqueous penicillin G, 2 million units IV or IM ½–1 hr before procedure and 1 million units IV or IM 6 hr after
C. Ampicillin, 2 gm IV or IM, plus gentamicin, 1.5 mg/kg IV or IM, ½ hr before procedure and 8 hr after*
D. Erythromycin, 1 gm PO 1 hr before procedure and 500 mg PO 6 hr after
E. Vancomycin, 1 gm IV (slowly over 1 hr) starting 1 hr before procedure
F. Amoxicillin, 3 gm PO 1 hr before procedure and 1.5 gm PO 6 hr after
G. Vancomycin, 1 gm IV (slowly over 1 hr), plus gentamicin, 1.5 mg/kg IV or IM, 1 hr before procedure and 8 hr after
H. Cefazolin, 1 gm IV ½ hr before procedure and q6h × 4 doses after
I. Ampicillin, 2 gm IV or IM, plus gentamicin, 1.5 mg/kg IV or IM, ½ hr before procedure and 8 hr after

Type of procedure	Predisposing condition
Congenital, rheumatic, and acquired heart disease (except uncomplicated secundum atrial septal defect), idiopathic hypertrophic subaortic stenosis, mitral valve prolapse syndrome	Prosthetic heart valve, previous endocarditis, continuous oral penicillin prophylaxis for rheumatic fever, surgical systemic-pulmonary shunt

	A, B	C
Dental procedures, surgery, or instrumentation of upper respiratory tract	Penicillin-allergic patients: D	Penicillin-allergic patients: E
Surgery or instrumentation of gastrointestinal or genitourinary tract	F (minor procedures) I (others) Penicillin-allergic patients: G	I Penicillin-allergic patients: G
Cardiovascular surgery, vascular prosthesis	H or E	G

*Penicillin V, 1 gm PO 6 hr after procedure, may be substituted for ampicillin/gentamicin 8 hr after procedure

References

1. Weinstein L: Infectious Endocarditis. In general reference 7, p 1127.
2. Prevention of Bacterial Endocarditis. *Medical Letter* 29(754):109, 1987.
3. Kaye D: Prophylaxis for Infective Endocarditis: An Update. *Ann Intern Med* 104:419, 1986.

3-B. Isoniazid Prophylaxis of Tuberculous Infection*

Eligible persons are listed by priority grouping:

1. Household members and others in close contact with an infectious case.†
2. Positive tuberculin reactors who have chest x-ray findings characteristic of inactive tuberculous infection with a life expectancy of greater than 10 years
3. Recent tuberculin skin-test converters (i.e., skin test induration has increased by at least 6 mm from less than 10 mm to more than 10 mm in less than 24 mo)
4. Positive tuberculin reactors who have any of the following conditions:
   a. Chronic corticosteroid or immunosuppressive therapy
   b. Chronic malignancy, especially lymphoma
   c. Silicosis
   d. Diabetes mellitus
   e. Postgastrectomy or malnutrition
   f. Chronic renal failure
   g. Acquired immunodeficiency syndrome (AIDS)
5. Positive tuberculin reactors under age 35 who have never received isoniazid prophylaxis

References
1. American Thoracic Society, Medical Section of the American Lung Association: Treatment of Tuberculosis and other Mycobacterial Disease. *Am Rev Respir Dis* 127:790, 1983.
2. Daniel TM: Tuberculosis. In general reference 1, p 632.

*Before isoniazid chemoprophylaxis is begun, it is essential to exclude active infection (for which single-drug therapy is inadequate).
†Treatment can be stopped if a skin test after 3 months of therapy is negative.

3-C. Guidelines for Tetanus Prophylaxis

History of Tetanus Immunization (Doses)	Clean Minor Wound		All Other Wounds	
	Toxoid[a]	Antitoxin[b]	Toxoid	Antitoxin
Uncertain	Yes	No	Yes	Yes
None	Yes	No	Yes	Yes
< 3	Yes	No	Yes	Yes[c]
≥ 3	No[d]	No	No[e]	No

[a] Adult-type tetanus and diphtheria toxoids (Td) for patients > 6 yr old.
[b] Human tetanus immune globulin (TIG) is preferred given as 250 units IM.
[c] Except if at least 2 doses of toxoid are given and wound is < 24 hr old.
[d] Unless more than 10 yr since last dose.
[e] Unless more than 5 yr since last dose.

References
1. Beaty HN: Tetanus. In general reference 1, p. 560.
2. Furste W: Four Keys to 100 Percent Success in Tetanus Prophylaxis. *Am J Surg* 128:616, 1974.

3-D. Selected Venereal Diseases: Current Treatment Recommendations

Gonorrhea

Diagnosis	Recommended treatment
Uncomplicated gonococcal infection in men and women	Amoxicillin, 3.0 gm PO; or ampicillin, 3.5 gm PO; or aqueous procaine penicillin G (APPG), 4.8 million units IM; or ceftriaxone, 250 mg IM
	Amoxicillin, ampicillin, and penicillin (but not ceftriaxone) are accompanied by probenecid, 1 gm PO (APPG may be less desirable because of associated pain and toxicity)
	PLUS
	Tetracycline HCl, 500 mg PO qid for 7 days; or doxycycline, 100 mg PO bid for 7 days
	OR
	For patients in whom tetracyclines are contraindicated or not tolerated, the single-dose regimen may be followed by erythromycin base or stearate, 500 mg PO qid for 7 days, or erythromycin ethylsuccinate, 800 mg PO qid for 7 days
Anorectal infection in men	Procaine penicillin G, 4.8 million units IM, with probenecid, 1 gm PO; or ceftriaxone, 250 mg IM
	If allergic to penicillin: spectinomycin, 2.0 gm IM

Pharyngeal infection

Ceftriaxone, 250 mg IM; or procaine penicillin, 4.8 million units, divided between two sites, with probenecid, 1 gm PO
If allergic to penicillins and cephalosporins: trimethoprim-sulfamethoxazole, 9 single-strength tablets qd for 5 days

Treatment failures or infection with penicillinase-producing Neisseria gonorrhoeae

Spectinomycin, 2.0 gm IM; or ceftriaxone, 250 mg IM

Gonococcal infection in pregnancy

Amoxicillin, 3.0 gm PO; or ampicillin, 3.5 gm PO; or ceftriaxone, 250 mg IM; consider adding a tetracycline or doxycycline oral regimen for Chlamydia infection
Aqueous procaine penicillin G, 4.8 million units IM, is effective but is less desirable because of associated pain and toxicity
Amoxicillin, ampicillin, and penicillin (but not ceftriaxone) are accompanied by probenecid, 1 gm PO
If allergic to penicillins and cephalosporins: spectinomycin, 2 gm IM

Acute salpingitis (pelvic inflammatory disease)
Outpatients

PLUS
Erythromycin base, 500 mg; or erythromycin ethylsuccinate, 800 mg PO qid for 7 days
Cefoxitin, 2 gm IM

OR

Ampicillin, 3.5 gm PO; or amoxicillin, 3.0 gm PO; or procaine penicillin, 4.8 million units IM; each with probenecid, 1 gm PO, followed by doxycycline 100 mg bid for 10–14 days
Ceftriaxone, 250 IM, without probenecid is also effective

Gonorrhea (continued)

Diagnosis	Recommended treatment
Hospitalized patients (at least 4 days of IV and 14 days of total therapy)	Doxycycline, 100 mg IV q12h; cefoxitin, 2 gm IV q6h; followed by doxycycline, 100 mg bid PO OR Clindamycin, 600 mg IV q6h; gentamicin, 1.5 mg/kg IV q8h in patients with normal renal function; followed by clindamycin, 450 mg PO q12h OR Doxycycline, 100 mg IV q12h; metronidazole, 500 mg IV q6h for at least 4 days; followed by both drugs, same dosage, PO for 14-day total course
Disseminated gonococcal infection (arthritis/dermatitis syndrome)	Aqueous crystalline penicillin G, 10 million units/day IV for at least 3 days; followed by amoxicillin or ampicillin, 500 mg PO qid to complete at least 7 days of therapy OR Amoxicillin, 3.0 gm PO; or ampicillin, 3.5 gm PO; each with probenecid, 1.0 gm PO, followed by amoxicillin or ampicillin, 500 mg PO qid for at least 7 days

OR

Cefoxitin, 1.0 gm IV qid for at least 7 days

OR

Cefotaxime, 500 mg IV qid for at least 7 days

OR

Ceftriaxone, 1 gm IV qd for 7 days

Tetracycline, 0.5 gm PO qid for 7 days; or doxycycline, 100 mg bid for 7 days; or erythromycin, 0.5 gm PO qid for 7–14 days

Nongonococcal urethritis

Syphilis

Diagnosis	Recommended treatment	
	Non-penicillin-allergic	Penicillin-allergic
Primary, secondary, or early latent	Benzathine penicillin, G, 2.4 million units IM (half in each hip) as single dose OR Procaine penicillin G, 600,000 units IM qd for 8 days	Erythromycin or tetracycline, 0.5 gm PO qid for 15 days
Late latent or latent of undetermined duration	Benzathine penicillin G, 2.4 million units IM once a week for 3 weeks (7.2 million units total)	Erythromycin or tetracycline, 0.5 gm PO qid for 30 days
Neurosyphilis	Penicillin G, 2–4 million units IV q4h for 10 days; or penicillin G procaine, 2.4 million units IM qd, and probenecid, 500 mg PO qid, both for 10 days PLUS	Erythromycin or tetracycline, 0.5 gm PO qid for 30 days

Late cardiovascular or benign tertiary	Penicillin G benzathine, 2.4 million units IM once a week for 3 weeks	Erythromycin or tetracycline, 0.5 gm PO qid for 30 days
	Benzathine penicillin G, 2.4 million units IM once a week for 3 weeks	

References
1. 1985 STD Treatment Guidelines. *MMWR* 34:815, 1985.
2. Holmes KK, Morse SA: Gonococcal Infections. In general reference 19, p 580.
3. Rudolph AH: Syphilis. In general reference 19, p 611.
4. U.S. Department of Health, Education, and Welfare. Public Health Service, Center for Disease Control: Gonorrhea: Center for Disease Control Recommended Treatment Schedules, 1979. *Ann Intern Med* 90:809, 1979.
5. Syphilotherapy 1976: Position Paper for the Current USPHS Recommendations. *J Am Vener Dis Assoc* 3:98, 1976.
6. Treatment of Sexually Transmitted Diseases. *Medical Letter* 30(757):5, 1988.

3-E. Common Drugs Requiring Dosage Adjustment in Renal Failure

Antibiotics
Acyclovir
Amantadine
Aminoglycosides (e.g., tobramycin)
Amphotericin
Aztreonam
Cephalosporins (except cefoperazone, ceftriaxone)
Ciprofloxacin
Cycloserine
Doxycycline
Erythromycin
Ethambutol
5-Fluorocytosine
Imipenem
Isoniazid (especially slow acetylators)
Metronidazole
Nalidixic acid
Nitrofurantoin
Norfloxacin
Penicillins (except cloxacillin, dicloxacillin, nafcillin, oxacillin)
Pentamidine
Sulfamethoxazole-trimethroprim
Sulfisoxazole
Tetracylines (except minocycline)
Vancomycin

Analgesics
Acetaminophen
Aspirin
Methadone
Phenazopyridine (Pyridium)
Propoxyphene (Darvon)

Sedatives
Chlordiazepoxide (Librium)
Chloral hydrate
Ethchlorvynol
Glutethimide (Doriden)
Lithium carbonate
Meprobamate
Methaqualone
Midazolam
Phenobarbital

Cardiovascular Drugs
Acebutolol
Acetazolamide
Amiloride
Atenolol
Bretylium
Captopril
Clonidine
Chlorthalidone
Digitoxin (for creatinine clearance < 10 ml/min)
Digoxin
Disopyramide (Norpace)
Enalapril
Encainide
Flecainide
Guanethidine
Hydralazine
Methyldopa
Metoprolol
Mexiletine
Nadolol
Nitroprusside
Procainamide
Spironolactone
Tocainide
Triamterene
Verapamil

Antineoplastic and Immunosuppressive Drugs
Adriamycin
Azathioprine
Bleomycin
Cisplatin
Cyclophosphamide
Hydroxyurea
Melphalan
Methotrexate
Mithramycin
Mitomycin C
Nitrosourea
Streptozotocin

Arthritic Drugs
Allopurinol
Colchicine
Diflunisal
Gold
Ibuprofen (Motrin)

Naproxen
Phenylbutazone
Probenecid
Sulfinpyrazone
Sulindac

Anticonvulsants
Carbamazepine (Tegretol)
Ethosuximide
Primidone
Phenobarbital

Miscellaneous Agents
Baclofen
Cimetidine
Clofibrate
Cyclosporine
Diphenhydramine (Benadryl)
Gallamine (Flaxedil)
Gemfibrozil
Hypoglycemic agents
  Insulin
  Chlorpropamide (Diabinese)
  Acetohexamide (Dymelor)
  Tolbutamide (Orinase)
Magnesium antacids
Metoclopramide
Nicotinic acid
Pancuronium
Propylthiouracil
Ranitidine
Terbutaline (especially parenteral)

Reference
1. Bennett WM, Muther RS, Parker RA, et al: Drug Therapy in Renal Failure: Dosing Guidelines for Adults. *Ann Intern Med* 93:62, 286, 1980.
2. Bennett WM, Aronoff GR, Golper PA, et al: *Drug Prescribing in Renal Failure.* Philadelphia: American College of Physicians, 1987.

3-F. Guidelines for Intravenous Aminophylline Therapy*

Loading dose[a]

	Dose (mg/kg)[b]
No known theophylline ingestion in past 24–48 hr	5–6 mg/kg over 15–30 min
Theophylline ingested within past 48 hr	0–3 mg/kg over 15–30 min
Poor clinical response to initial loading dose and no clinical signs of toxicity, or theophylline blood level < 15 μg/ml	Additional 1–3 mg/kg over 15–30 min

[a]To achieve a serum level of 10 μg/ml from 0 μg/ml.
[b]Based on ideal body weight.

Maintenance dose (continuous infusion)

	Dose (mg/kg/hr)[a]
Children > 9 yr old and adult smokers < 55 yr old	0.50–0.90
Adult nonsmokers	0.60
Severe airway obstruction	0.40
Mild-to-moderate heart failure	≤0.40
Severe heart failure	≤0.20
Pneumonia	0.20–0.40
Liver dysfunction with serum bilirubin < 1.5 mg/dl and serum albumin > 2.9 gm/dl	≤0.45
Liver dysfunction with serum bilirubin > 1.5 mg/dl and/or serum albumin < 2.9 gm/dl	≤0.20

[a]Patients taking propranolol, erythromycin, cimetidine, diltiazem, or quinolones metabolize theophylline more slowly and may require a reduction in dosage. Patients taking phenytoin, phenobarbital, or rifampin may require an increase in dosage.

References
1. Hendeles L, Weinberger M: Poisoning Patients with Intravenous Theophylline (editorial). *Am J Hosp Pharm* 37:49, 1980.
2. Powell JR, Vozeh S, Hopewell P, et al: Theophylline Disposition in Acutely Ill Hospitalized Patients. *Am Rev Respir Dis* 118:229, 1978.
3. Hendeles L, Weinberger M, Bighley L: Disposition of Theophylline after a Single Intravenous Infusion of Aminophylline. *Am Rev Respir Dis* 118:97, 1978.

*Serum theophylline determinations after 12 to 36 hr of continuous aminophylline infusion are useful.

3-G. Dopamine and Dobutamine Dosage Charts

Dopamine (Intropin) 800 mg (4 vials)/500 ml = 1.6 mg/ml

Weight		Dosage (µg/kg/min)*							
lb	kg	1.0	2.5	5.0	7.5	10.0	12.5	15.0	20.0
88	40	2	4	7	11	15	19	22	30
99	45	2	4	8	12	17	20	25	34
110	50	2	5	9	14	19	23	28	38
121	55	2	5	10	15	22	25	31	42
132	60	3	6	11	17	23	28	34	46
143	65	3	6	12	18	25	30	36	49
154	70	4	7	13	20	26	33	39	52
165	75	4	7	14	21	28	35	42	57
176	80	4	8	15	22	30	38	45	60
187	85	4	8	16	23	32	40	48	64
198	90	4	9	17	25	34	42	51	68
209	95	5	9	18	26	36	45	53	72
220	100	5	10	19	27	38	47	57	76

*Flow rate in drops/min; based on a microdrip: 60 drops = 1 ml.
Source: Freitag JJ, Miller LW (Eds): *Manual of Medical Therapeutics* (23rd ed). Boston: Little, Brown, 1980, app IV, p 455.

Dobutamine (Dobutrex) 500 mg (2 vials)/500 ml = 1.0 mg/ml

Weight		Dosage (μg/kg/min)*							
lb	kg	1.0	2.5	5.0	7.5	10.0	12.5	15.0	20.0
88	40	2	5	11	16	22	29	36	45
99	45	3	7	14	20	27	34	41	54
110	50	3	8	15	23	30	38	45	60
121	55	3	8	17	25	33	41	50	66
132	60	4	9	18	27	36	45	54	72
143	65	4	10	20	29	39	49	59	78
154	70	4	11	21	32	42	53	63	84
165	75	5	11	23	34	45	56	68	90
176	80	5	12	24	36	48	60	72	96
187	85	5	13	26	38	51	64	77	102
198	90	5	14	27	41	54	68	81	108
209	95	6	14	29	43	57	71	86	114
220	100	6	15	30	45	60	75	90	120

*Flow rate in drops/min; based on a microdrip; 60 drops = 1 ml.
Source: Freitag JJ, Miller LW (Eds): *Manual of Medical Therapeutics* (23rd ed). Boston: Little, Brown, 1980, app V, p 456.

3-H. Glucocorticoid Preparations

USP name	Trade name	Tablet size (mg)	Relative anti-inflam-matory potency	Relative mineralo-corticoid potency	Approximate equivalent dose (mg)	Biologic half-life (hr)[a]
Short-acting						
Hydrocortisone (cortisol)	Cortef, Solu-Cortef[b]	5, 10, 20	1.0	1.0	20.0	8–12
Cortisone		5, 10, 20	0.8	0.8	25.0	8–12
Intermediate-acting						
Prednisone	Deltasone, Meticorten	1, 2.5, 5, 10, 20, 50	4.0	0.8	5.0	12–36
Prednisolone	Delta-Cortef, Meticortelone	5	4.0	0.8	5.0	12–36
Methylprednisolone	Medrol, Solu-Medrol[b]	2, 4, 8, 16, 24, 32	5.0	0.5	4.0	12–36
Triamcinolone	Aristocort, Kenacort	1, 2, 4, 8, 16	5.0	0	4.0	12–36

3-H. Glucocorticoid Preparations (continued)

USP name	Trade name	Tablet size (mg)	Relative anti-inflammatory potency	Relative mineralocorticoid potency	Approximate equivalent dose	Biologic half-life (hr)[a]
Long-acting						
Dexamethasone	Decadron, Hexadrol	0.25, 0.5, 0.75, 1.5, **4**	25	0	0.75	36–72
Betamethasone	Celestone	0.6	25	0	0.60	36–72

[a]Apply to only oral and intravenous routes of administration.
[b]parenteral form.
Source: Modified from Kaine JL: Arthritis and Rheumatologic Diseases. In general reference 2, p 379.

References

1. Haynes RC, Murad F: Adrenocorticotropic Hormone, Adrenocortical Steroids and Their Synthetic Analogs; Inhibitors of Adrenocortical Steroid Biosynthesis. In Gilman AG, Goodman LS, Rall TW, Murad F (Eds): *The Pharmacological Basis of Therapeutics* (7th ed). New York: Macmillan, 1985, p 1475.
2. Axelrod L: Glucocorticoid Therapy. *Medicine* 55:39, 1976.

3-I. Hypoglycemic Agents

Characteristics of commonly used insulin preparations

Classification	Insulin preparation	Onset	Peak	Duration (hr)
Rapid-acting	Regular	IV: immediate IM: 5–30 min SC: 15–60 min	15–30 min 30–60 min 2–6 hr	2 2–4 4–12
	Semilente	SC: 30–60 min	3–6 hr	8–16
Intermediate-acting	NPH	SC: 1.5–4 hr	6–16 hr	12–24
	Lente	SC: 1–4 hr	6–16 hr	12–28
Slow-acting	Protamine zinc insulin (PZI)	SC: 3–8 hr	14–24 hr	24–48
	Ultralente	SC: 3–8 hr	14–24 hr	24–48

Source: Modified from Orland MJ: Diabetes Mellitus. In general reference 2, p 321.

Oral hypoglycemic agents (sulfonylureas)*

Type	Available form (mg)	Total daily dose (mg)	Duration of action (hr)	Dose given
Tolbutamide (Orinase)	250, 500	500–3000	6–12	bid–tid
Chlorpropamide (Diabinese)	100, 250	100–500	up to 90	qd–bid
Acetohexamide (Dymelor)	250, 500	250–1500	12–24	qd–tid
Tolazamide (Tolinase)	100, 250, 500	100–1000	12–24	qd–bid
Glipizide (Glucotrol)	5, 10	5–40	12–24	qd–bid
Glyburide (DiaBeta, Micronase)	1.25, 2.5, 5	2.5–20	24–60	qd–bid

*Phenformin drugs have been removed from the market by the FDA.
Source: Modified from Orland MJ: Diabetes Mellitus. In general reference 2, p. 320.

Factors Causing Hyperglycemia in Diabetics
Weight gain or increased carbohydrate ingestion
Intravenous carbohydrate infusion (e.g., hyperalimentation)
Pubertal growth
Nonuse or incorrect use of insulin
Infection or inflammation
Ketoacidosis
Other acute stress (e.g., myocardial infarction, pancreatitis,
    surgery)
Endocrinopathies
  Hyperthyroidism
  Pheochromocytoma
  Hyperadrenocorticism
  Profound hyperlipidemia
  Primary hyperparathyroidism
  Acromegaly
Decreased activity
Pancreatic disease or resection
Hypokalemia
Drugs
  Nicotinic acid
  Diazoxide
  Glucocorticoids
  Phenytoin
  Thyroid hormone preparations
  Diuretics
  Oral contraceptives
Change in oral hypoglycemic therapy
Insulin or insulin-receptor antibodies
Insulin-resistant states

Factors Causing Hypoglycemia in Diabetics
Weight reduction or decreased carbohydrate ingestion
Decreased intravenous carbohydrate infusion
Increased activity
Drug interactions with sulfonylurea therapy
  Warfarin
  Salicylates
  Chloramphenicol
  Clofibrate
  Sulfonamides
  Methyldopa
  Phenylbutazone
  Monoamine oxidase inhibitors
Renal insufficiency
Alcohol ingestion
Hypothyroidism
Hypoadrenocorticism

Decreased dosage or discontinuation of drugs (e.g., glucocorticoids, diuretics, thyroid hormone preparations)
Intercurrent processes causing hypoglycemia (see 4-J)

References
1. Garber AJ: Diabetes Mellitus. In Stein JH (Ed): *Internal
   Medicine* (2nd ed). Boston: Little, Brown, 1983, p 1997.
2. Foster DW: Diabetes Mellitus. In general reference 1, p
   1778.

3-J. Selected Intravenous Vasoactive Drugs

Drug	Common preparations	Dosage	Comments
Dopamine (Intropin)	1 amp = 200 mg; add 2–4 amps to 250–500 ml 5% D/W	Initial dose: 1–4 µg/kg/min; titrate to effect	Doses > 12–14 µg/kg/min cause primarily alpha-adrenergic effects (e.g., vasoconstriction); doses < 10 µg/kg/min cause mainly beta-adrenergic effects (e.g., increased stroke volume) and increased renal blood flow
Dobutamine (Dobutrex)	1 amp = 250 mg; add 1–4 amps to 250–500 ml 5% D/W	Initial dose: 1–4 µg/kg/min; titrate to effect	Doses > 20 µg/kg/min may be associated with arrhythmias
Isoproterenol (Isuprel)	1 amp = 1 mg; add 1–2 amp to 500 ml 5% D/W	Initial dose: 1 µg/min; titrate to effect	Doses > 10 µg/min may be associated with arrhythmias
Levarterenol (Levophed)	1 amp = 8 mg; add 1–2 amps to 250–500 ml 5% D/W	Initial dose: 10–15 µg/min; titrate to effect	Mainly alpha-adrenergic effects (i.e., vasoconstriction) in most vascular beds

3-J. Selected Intravenous Vasoactive Drugs (continued)

Drug	Common preparations	Dosage	Comments
Amrinone (Inocor)	Dilute to 1–3 mg/ml concentration in saline solution. Do not use dextrose	Initial dose: 0.75 mg/kg over 2–3 min and then infuse continuously 5–10 µg/kg/min	Side effects: thrombocytopenia, gastrointestinal upset, fever, myalgia, hepatic dysfunction, ventricular irritability, and hypotension
Nitroprusside (Nipride)	1 amp = 50 mg; add 1–2 amps to 250 ml 5% D/W	Initial dose: 0.5–5 µg/kg/min; titrate to effect	Infusion apparatus must be shielded from light; infusion pump is required; total dose > 3 mg/kg may be associated with toxicity, especially when renal insufficiency is present

| Nitroglycerin | Variable, follow suppliers' recommendations | Initial dose: 5–10 μg/min. Increase by 5–10 μg/min every 3–5 min until response seen. Maximum dose: 200 μg/min | Use glass bottles and non-absorbing tubing. Treat hypotension with volume and cessation of infusion |

References

1. Shafer KE: Heart Failure. In general reference 2, p 99.
2. Jaffe AS: Cardiac Arrest and CPR. In general reference 2, p 146.
3. Weil MH, Planta MV, Rackow EC: Acute Circulatory Failure (Shock). In general reference 7, p 561.

3-K. Drug and Disease Interactions with Warfarin (Coumadin)

Increased Prothrombin Time
Acetaminophen
Age
Alcohol*
Allopurinol
Amiodarone
Anabolic steroids
Antibiotics
Bretylium
Chloral hydrate*
Chlorpropamide
Cholestyramine*
Chymotrypsin
Cimetidine
Clofibrate
Congestive heart failure
Danazol
Dextran
Dextrothyroxine
Diazoxide
Diflunisal
Disulfiram
Diuretics*
Erythromycin
Ethacrynic acid
Fever
Gemfibrozil
Glucagon
Guanethidine
Heparin
Hepatic disease
Hepatotoxic drugs
Hyperthyroidism
Hypoglycemic agents
Indomethacin
Influenza vaccine
Inhalation anesthetics
Ketoconazole
Mefenamic acid
Mercaptopurine
Methotrexate
Methyldopa
Methylphenidate

Metronidazole
Miconazole
Monoamine oxidase inhibitors
Nalidixic acid
Naproxen
Narcotics
Oxolinic acid
Oxyphenbutazone
Phenylbutazone
Phenytoin
Propoxyphene
Propranolol
Propylthiouracil
Pyrazolones
Quinidine
Quinine
Ranitidine
Reserpine
Salicylates (> 1 gm daily)
Sulfinpyrazone
Sulfonamides
Sulindac
Thyroid preparations
Tolbutamide
Triclofos sodium
Tricyclic antidepressants
Trimethoprim-sulfamethoxazole
Vitamin E
Vitamin K malabsorption or deficiency

Decreased Prothrombin Time
Alcohol*
Aluminum hydroxide
Antihistamines
Barbiturates
Carbamazepine
Chloral hydrate*
Chlordiazepoxide
Cholestyramine*
Colestipol
Diuretics*
Estrogens
Ethchlorvynol
Glutethimide
Griseofulvin
Haloperidol
Hereditary resistance

Insecticides
Meprobamate
Myxedema
Nafcillin
Nephrotic syndrome
Oral contraceptives
Paraldehyde
Pregnancy (mother only)
Primidone
Ranitidine
Rifampin
Simethicone
Sucralfate
Vitamin C
Vitamin K

References
1. *Physicians' Desk Reference.* Oradell, NJ: Medical Economics Co., 1987, p 897.
2. Tollefsen DM: Disorders of Hemostasis. In general reference 2, p 271.
3. O'Reilly RA: Anticoagulant, Antithrombotic and Thrombolytic Drugs. In Gilman AG, Goodman LS, Rall TW, Murad F (Eds): *The Pharmacological Basis of Therapeutics* (7th ed). New York: Macmillan, 1985, p 1347.

*Can cause increased or decreased prothrombin time.

4 ENDOCRINE/ METABOLIC SYSTEM

4-A. Amenorrhea

Hypothalamic and Pituitary Causes

Hypothalamic-pituitary dysfunction with hyperprolactinemia (see 4-C)
  Drugs (e.g., phenothiazines)
  Prolactinomas
  Primary hypothyroidism
Hypothalamic-pituitary dysfunction due to extrinsic factors
  Nutritional
    Obesity
    Weight loss (including anorexia nervosa)
  Strenuous exercise
  Stress
  Pseudocyesis
  Post-pill amenorrhea
  Chronic debilitating diseases (e.g., poorly-controlled diabetes mellitus, uremia, rheumatoid arthritis)
  Cushing's syndrome
  Late-onset congenital adrenal hyperplasia
  Lactation
  Pregnancy
Hypothalamic-pituitary dysfunction due to intrinsic factors
  Kallmann's syndrome

Empty sella syndrome
Hypopituitarism/hypothalamic disease (see 4-P)

Ovarian Causes
With decreased ovarian steroid production
  Congenital
    Gonadal agenesis
    Resistant ovary syndrome (Savage syndrome)
    Gonadal dysgenesis (including Turner's syndrome)
    Sex chromosome mosaicism
    XY gonadal dysgenesis
    17α-Hydroxylase deficiency
    True hermaphroditism
  Acquired: premature primary ovarian failure
    Autoimmune
    Chemotherapy
    Radiation
    Surgical castration
    Postinfection (e.g., mumps)
    Severe pelvic inflammatory disease
  Menopause
With increased ovarian steroid production
  Feminizing ovarian tumors
  Masculinizing ovarian tumors
  Polycystic ovary syndrome
  Chronic anovulation

Uterine and Outflow Tract Abnormalities
Hysterectomy
Müllerian agenesis
Müllerian anomalies
  Labial agglutination or fusion
  Imperforate hymen
  Absence or anomalies of vagina, cervix, or uterus
Trauma
  Cervical stenosis
  Vaginal stenosis
  Sclerosis of uterine cavity (Asherman's syndrome)
    Following postabortal or postpartum infection or
      trauma
    Following myomectomy or cesarean section
    Severe endometritis (including tuberculous endometri-
      tis)
Male pseudohermaphroditism
  Testicular feminization
  5th reductase deficiency

Female pseudohermaphroditism
   Congenital adrenal hyperplasia
   Exposure to maternal androgens in utero

References
1. Speroff L, Glass RH, Kase NG: *Clinical Gynecologic Endocrinology and Infertility.* Baltimore: Williams & Wilkins, 1983, p 141.
2. Jones HW, Jones GS (Eds): *Novak's Textbook of Gynecology.* Baltimore: William & Wilkins, 1981, p 733.

4-B. Gynecomastia

Pseudogynecomastia
   Obesity
   Benign or malignant breast tumor
Physiologic
   Newborn
   Adolescence
   Normal physical finding
   Old age
Familial gynecomastia
Persistent pubertal macromastia
Deficient testosterone production or action
   End organ insensitivity to androgens
      Testicular feminization
      Reifenstein's syndrome
   Primary hypogonadism
      Klinefelter's syndrome
      Congenital anorchia
      XX males
      Orchitis
         Viral
         Neisseria gonorrhoeae
         Granulomatous (especially leprosy)
      Irradiation
      Trauma
      Castration
      Associated with neurologic disease
         Myotonia atrophica
         Spinal cord disease
      Defects in testosterone synthesis
      Uremia

Secondary or tertiary hypogonadism (rarely)
  Kallmann's syndrome
  Hypopituitarism/hypothalamic disease (see 4-P)
Neoplasms
  Producing estrogens or estrogen precursors
    Feminizing adrenal tumors
    Testicular tumors
  Secreting human chorionic gonadotropin (HCG)
    Germinal cell tumors of the testicle
    Non-testicular tumors
      Gynecomastia reported with elevated HCG
        Undifferentiated mediastinal carcinoma
        Adenocarcinoma of the stomach
        Hepatoma, hepatoblastoma
        Carcinoma of the pancreas
        Carcinoma of the lung
      Detectable HCG reported without gynecomastia (so
        far)
        Lymphoma
        Melanoma
        Esophagus
        Biliary tract
        Small intestine
        Liver sarcoma
        Colon/rectal
        Leukemia
        Multiple myeloma
        Sarcomas
        Breast
        Insulinoma
        Pheochromocytoma
        Renal cell carcinoma
        Medullary carcinoma of the thyroid
  Secreting prolactin
    Pituitary prolactinomas
  Secreting gonadotropins
    Gonadotropin-secreting pituitary adenomas
Increased estrogen production
  True hermaphroditism
    Inherited increased peripheral aromatase activity
  Increased availability of estrogen precursors
    Liver disease (especially cirrhosis)
    Thyrotoxicosis
    Congenital adrenal hyperplasia
      11-Hydroxylase deficiency
      21-Hydroxylase deficiency

Systemic diseases (especially recovery from chronic disease)
  Refeeding gynecomastia (following starvation)
  Poorly controlled diabetes mellitus
  Pulmonary tuberculosis
Drugs
  Amphetamines
  Androgens
  Cimetidine
  Cyproterone
  Cytotoxic agents
    Busulfan
    Nitrosoureas
    Vincristine
    Combination chemotherapy
  Diazepam
  Diethylpropion
  Digitalis
  Estrogens
  Ethionamide
  Flutamide
  Gonadotropins
  Heroin
  Isoniazid
  Ketoconazole
  Marijuana
  Methyldopa
  Phenothiazines
  Phenytoin
  Reserpine
  Spironolactone
  Tricyclic antidepressants

References
1. Wilson JD, Aiman J, MacDonald PC: The Pathogenesis of Gynecomastia. *Adv Intern Med* 25:1, 1980.
2. Carlson HE: Gynecomastia. *N Engl J Med* 303:795, 1980.

4-C. Galactorrhea

Without hyperprolactinemia
  Pseudogalactorrhea
    Intramammary lesions
      Benign
        Fibrocystic disease
        Intraductal papilloma
      Malignant neoplasm
  Normal women who have been pregnant in the past
  Cushing's disease
  Hyperthyroidism
With hyperprolactinemia
  Drugs
    Neuroleptics
      Phenothiazines
      Thioxanthenes
      Butyrophenones
      Diphenylbutylpiperidines
      Dihydroindolones
    Reserpine
    Alpha-methyldopa
    Opiates
    Substituted benzamides
      Sulpiride
      Metoclopramide
      Celebropride
      Brompride
    Antidepressants
      Traditional tricyclic antidepressants
        Imipramine
        Desipramine
        Amitriptyline
        Nortriptyline
      Dibenzoxazepine antidepressants
        Amoxapine
    During or following withdrawal of estrogen/progestin
      combinations
    Cimetidine
    Verapamil
    Benzodiazepines
    Androgens
    Isoniazid
    Meprobamate
    Amphetamines
  Diseases affecting the hypothalamus and/or pituitary
    stalk

Central nervous sys
Craniopharyngioma
Pinealomas
Aneurysms
Hypothalamic tumor
Pituitary stalk sectio
   the stalk)
Encephalitis/postenc
Basilar meningitis
Pseudotumor cerebri
Post-pneumoenceph
Hydrocephalus
Neuraxis irradiation
Other destructive lesions of the hypothalamus (see
   4-P)
Tumors secreting prolactin or placental lactogen
  Prolactinomas
  Acromegaly
  Bronchogenic carcinoma
  Hypernephroma
  Chorionepithelioma
  Hydatidiform mole
Empty sella syndrome
Primary hypothyroidism
Pregnancy
Chronic renal failure
Refeeding after starvation
Addison's disease
Neural stimulation
  Disorders of the chest wall and thorax
    Thoracotomy
    Mastectomy/mammoplasty
    Thoracoplasty
    Burns
    Herpes zoster
    Bronchogenic tumors
    Bronchiectasis/chronic bronchitis
    Neoplasms of the chest wall
    Chest wall injury
  Nipple stimulation
    Chronic inflammatory disease
    Mechanical stimulation of the nipples
  Spinal cord
    Tabes dorsalis
    Syringomyelia
    Cervical spinal cord lesions
  Psychogenic
    Pseudocyesis

4-D. HYPOTHERMIA

Stresses
Posttrauma
Major surge
Idiopathic hyp

References
1. Kleinb
  Stu

and anesthesia
...rprolactinemia

...erg DL, Noel GC, Frantz AG: Galactorrhea: A
...dy of 235 Cases, Including 48 With Pituitary Tumors.
...Engl J Med 296:589, 1977.
2. Besser GM, Edwards CRW: Galactorrhea. *Br Med J*
2:280, 1972.
3. Tolis G, Somma M, Van Camperhaut J, et al: Prolactin
Secretion In 65 Patients With Galactorrhea. *Am J Obstet
Gynecol* 118:91, 1974.

4-D. Hypothermia

Accidental hypothermia
    Environmental exposure (especially in neonates, prema-
        ture or low-birth-weight babies, elderly, or persons
        who are unconscious, immobilized, drugged, or ex-
        hausted)
    Cold-water immersion
Endocrine disorders
    Hypothyroidism
    Hypoglycemia
    Adrenal insufficiency
    Hypopituitarism
    Diabetic ketoacidosis
Other systemic disorders (especially in the elderly coma-
    tose)
    Pancreatitis
    Uremia
    Hepatic failure
    Congestive heart failure
    Myocardial infarction
    Respiratory failure
Drugs
    Ethanol
    Barbiturates

Phenothiazines
General anesthesia
Hypothalamic and central nervous system dysfunction
Wernicke's encephalopathy
Cerebrovascular accidents
Head trauma
Brain tumors
Spinal cord transection above T1
Anorexia nervosa
Shapiro's syndrome
Spontaneous periodic hypothermia
Other hypothalamic lesions (e.g., sarcoidosis, infarction)
Dermal disorders
Burns
Erythrodermas
Sepsis
Protein-calorie malnutrition
Iatrogenic causes
Administration of cold blood or IV fluids
Iced saline gastric lavage
Peritoneal dialysis

References

1. Reuler JB: Hypothermia: Pathophysiology, Clinical Settings, and Management. *Ann Intern Med* 89:519, 1978.
2. Welton DE, Mattox KD, Miller RR, Petmecky FF: Treatment of Profound Hypothermia. *JAMA* 240:2291, 1978.
3. Petersdorf RG, Rott RK: Disorders of Heat Regulation. In general reference 1, p 48.

4-E. Weight Gain

Increased body fluid (see 2-B)
Exogenous obesity
Cushing's syndrome
Hypogonadism
Hypothyroidism
Insulinoma
Congenital diseases
  Pseudohypoparathyroidism
  Prader-Willi syndrome
  Börjeson syndrome
  Laurence-Moon-Biedl syndrome
  Bicmond syndrome
  Carpenter syndrome
Drugs
  Oral contraceptive use
  Pharmacologic doses of glucocorticoids
Disturbances of hypothalamic satiety centers
  Tumors
  Trauma
  Encephalitis
Acromegaly

References
1. Foster DW: Gain and Loss in Weight. In general reference 1, p 176.
2. Frohman LA, Felig P, Broadus AE, Baxter JD: The Clinical Manifestations of Endocrine Disease. In general reference 8, p 25.

4-F. Weight Loss

Endocrine disorders
  Diabetes mellitus
  Thyrotoxicosis
  Adrenal insufficiency
  Pheochromocytoma
  Panhypopituitarism
Gastrointestinal disease
  Decreased food intake
    Poor or absent teeth
    Oral disease

Esophageal disease
Reflux
Esophagitis
Stricture
Neoplasm
Neuromuscular dysfunction
Peptic ulcer
Maldigestion/malabsorption (see 6-G)
Inflammatory bowel disease
Parasitic infestation
Infection, especially:
Tuberculosis
Bacterial endocarditis
Fungal diseases
Amebic abscess
Chronic pleuropulmonary suppurative disease (e.g., empyema)
Malignancy, especially:
Gastrointestinal
Pancreatic
Pulmonary
Hepatic
Leukemia
Lymphoma
Psychiatric disease
Anorexia nervosa
Depression
Psychosis
Anxiety
Malnutrition
Severe chronic organ failure
Renal failure
Heart failure (cardiac cachexia)
Pulmonary disease
Hepatic disease

Reference
1. Foster DW: Gain and Loss In Weight. In general reference 1, p 157.

4-G. Adrenal Insufficiency

Primary
Idiopathic/autoimmune
Tuberculosis
Vascular
  Hemorrhage
    Sepsis
    Anticoagulants
    Coagulopathy
    Trauma
    Surgery
    Pregnancy
    Neonatal
  Infarction
    Thrombosis
    Embolism
    Arteritis
Fungal infection
  Histoplasmosis
  Coccidioidomycosis
  Blastomycosis
  Moniliasis
  Torulopsosis
  Cryptococcosis
Infiltrative
  Hemochromatosis
  Sarcoidosis
  Amyloidosis
Neoplastic
  Lymphoma
  Metastatic cancer
  Leukemic infiltration
Iatrogenic
  Irradiation
  Bilateral adrenalectomy
Drugs
  Enzyme inhibitors
    Metyrapone
    Aminoglutethimide
    Trilostane
  Cytotoxic
Congenital/genetic
  Adrenoleukodystrophy
  Congenital adrenal hyperplasia
  Adrenal hypoplasia/aplasia

Familial glucocorticoid deficiency (hereditary unrespon-
siveness to adrenocorticotropic hormone [ACTH])

Secondary (Pituitary) or Tertiary (Hypothalamic)
Pituitary/hypothalamic lesions (see 4-P)
Isolated ACTH deficiency
Glucocorticoid therapy
Following removal of cortisol-secreting adrenal tumor

Reference
1. Baxter JD, Tyrrell JB: The Adrenal Cortex. In general reference 8, p 581.

4-H. Diabetes Insipidus

Nephrogenic (see 7-B)
Central
  Idiopathic
    Familial
    Sporadic
  Traumatic
    Head injury (basilar skull fracture)
    Birth trauma
  Iatrogenic
    Surgery
    Irradiation
  Infection
    Basilar meningitis
    Encephalitis
    Measles
    Mumps
    Diphtheria
    Scarlet fever
    Landry-Guillain-Barré syndrome
    Brain abscess
    Tuberculosis
    Brucellosis
    Actinomycosis
    Syphilis

Vascular
  Infarction (Sheehan's syndrome)
  Hemorrhage
  Thrombosis
  Aneurysm
  Vasculitis
  Sickle cell disease
Neoplasm
  Glioma
  Craniopharyngioma
  Astrocytoma
  Pinealoma
  Meningioma
  Leukemia
  Lymphoma
  Metastatic cancer (especially breast)
Infiltrative
  Amyloidosis
  Histiocytosis X
  Eosinophilic granuloma
  Sarcoidosis
Miscellaneous
  Collagen vascular disease
  Fat embolus
  Suprasellar and intrasellar cysts
  Anorexia nervosa

References
1. Coe FL: Alterations in Urinary Function. In general reference 1, p 194.
2. Thomas WC: Diabetes Insipidus. *J Clin Endocrinol Metab* 17:565, 1957.
3. Coggins CH, Reof A: Diabetes Insipidus. *Am J Med* 42:807, 1967.

4-I. Hyperglycemia

Inadequate dietary preparation for glucose tolerance test
Spontaneous diabetes mellitus
    Type I (insulin dependent)
    Type II (non–insulin dependent)
Secondary diabetes mellitus
    Pancreatic disease
        Chronic pancreatitis
        Pancreatectomy
        Pancreatic carcinoma
        Hemochromatosis
        Cystic fibrosis
    Hormonal abnormalities
        Increased counterregulatory hormones due to stress
            Infection
            Myocardial infarction
            Stroke
            Renal insufficiency
            Hepatic insufficiency
        Acromegaly
        Cushing's syndrome
        Pheochromocytoma
        Glucagonoma
        Hyperthyroidism
    Drug-induced
        Glucocorticoids
        Estrogens, including oral contraceptives
        Thiazides and loop diuretics
        Phenytoin
        Salicylates
        Nicotinic acid
        Chlorpromazine
        Diazoxide
        Growth hormone
        Indomethacin
    Insulin receptor abnormalities
    Associated with complex genetic syndromes
        Ataxia-telangiectasia
        Laurence-Moon-Biedl syndrome
        Myotonic dystrophy
        Friedreich's ataxia
        The lipodystrophies
Impaired glucose tolerance
Gestational diabetes

***Factors Causing Worsening of Compensated
Diabetes (see also 3-I)***
Increased caloric intake
Weight gain
Decreased exercise
Infection
Trauma
Surgery
Stroke
Pregnancy
Myocardial infarction

Reference

1. Felig P: The Endocrine Pancreas: Diabetes Mellitus. In
   general reference 8, p 1093.

4-J. Hypoglycemia

Fasting
Overutilization of glucose
  Insulin excess
    Pancreatic beta-cell disorders
      Insulinoma
      Islet-cell hyperplasia
      Nesidioblastosis
      Adenomatosis
      Beckwith's syndrome
      Leprechaunism
    Insulin autoimmune hypoglycemia
    Neonatal hypoglycemia (diabetic mother)
    Erythroblastosis fetalis
  Extrapancreatic tumors
    Bulky mesenchymal tumors
    Hepatomas
    Adrenocortical carcinomas
    Mesotheliomas
    Gastrointestinal carcinomas
    Lymphomas
    Other (kidney, ovary, lung)
  Systemic carnitine deficiency

Underproduction of glucose
  Inborn errors of glycogen metabolism
  Disorders of gluconeogenesis
  Severe hepatic dysfunction
    Acute fulminant hepatic necrosis
      Toxins
        Carbon tetrachloride
        Yellow phosphorus
        Chloroform
        Glycol
        Halothane
      Viral hepatitis
    Fatty liver of pregnancy
    Neoplasia (rare)
    Cirrhosis (rare)
    Congestive heart failure
  Deficiencies of insulin counterregulatory hormones
    Growth hormone deficiency (children)
    Adrenal insufficiency
    Glucagon deficiency
    Hypothyroidism
    Hypopituitarism
  Substrate deficiency
    Fasting hypoglycemia of pregnancy (late)
    Ketotic hypoglycemia of infancy
    Uremia
    Severe malnutrition
    Ackee fruit ingestion
  Idiopathic hypoglycemia of infancy and childhood
  Drug-induced hypoglycemia
    Insulin (iatrogenic or factitious)
    Sulfonylureas and phenformin (iatrogenic or factitious)
    Salicylates
    Ethanol
    Propranolol
    Pentamidine
    Sulfonamides
    Chloramphenicol
    Oxytetracycline
    Phenylbutazone
    Coumarin derivatives
    Probenecid
    Haloperidol
    Chlorpromazine
    Anabolic steroids
    Monoamine oxidase inhibitors

Reactive
Induced by glucose
    Alimentary
        Partial or total gastrectomy
        Pyloroplasty
        Gastrojejunostomy
        Peptic ulcer disease
    Functional/idiopathic
    Early type II diabetes mellitus
    Endocrine deficiencies
        Adrenal insufficiency
        Hypothyroidism
Induced by other substrates
    Galactosemia
    Hereditary fructose intolerance
    Familial leucine hypersensitivity

References
1. Cryer PE: Glucose Homeostasis and Hypoglycemia. In general reference 9, p 999.
2. Sherwin RS, Felig P: Hypoglycemia. In general reference 8, p 1182.
3. Foster DW, Rubenstein AH: Hypoglycemia, Insulinoma, and Other Hormone-Secreting Tumors of the Pancreas. In general reference 1, p 1800.

4-K. Hyperlipidemias

Type I (chylomicrons)
  Primary
    Familial lipoprotein lipase deficiency
    Familial apolipoprotein C-II deficiency
    Inherited circulating lipoprotein lipase inhibitor
  Secondary
    Dysglobulinemias (lupus, myeloma, lymphoma, Waldenström's)
    Hypothyroidism
    Severe diabetes mellitus
    Oral contraceptives
    High-dose glucocorticoids
    Glycogen storage disease
Type IIA (low-density lipoproteins [LDL]) and IIB (LDL + very low-density lipoproteins [VLDL])
  Primary
    Familial hypercholesterolemia
      Deficiency of LDL receptors
      Defective LDL receptors
      LDL internalization defect
    Familial combined hyperlipidemia
  Secondary
    IIA and IIB
      Nephrotic syndrome
      Biliary obstruction
      Pregnancy
      Hypothyroidism
      Glucocorticoids
      Cushing's syndrome
      Werner's syndrome
    IIA only
      Hepatoma
      Excess dietary cholesterol
      Acute intermittent porphyria
      Anorexia nervosa
      Dysglobulinemias
Type III (intermediate-density lipoproteins)
  Primary
    Apolipoprotein E2 homozygotes
    Other apolipoprotein E variants
    Apolipoprotein E deficiency
    Hepatic lipase deficiency
  Secondary
    Hypothyroidism
    Diabetes mellitus

      Alcohol
      Dysglobulinemias
      Liver disease

Type IV (VLDL)
  Primary
    Familial hypertriglyceridemia
    Familial combined hyperlipidemia
    Sporadic hypertriglyceridemia
  Secondary
    Alcohol
    Nephrotic syndrome
    Diabetes mellitus
    Hypothyroidism
    Pancreatitis
    Uremia
    Glucocorticoids
    Cushing's syndrome
    Dysglobulinemias
    Oral contraceptives
    Type I glycogenosis
    Obesity
    Pregnancy
    Stress
    Thiazides
    Beta-adrenergic blockers
    Growth hormone excess
    Congenital lipodystrophy

Type V (VLDL and chylomicrons)
  Primary
    Familial hypertriglyceridemia (severe form)
      Apolipoprotein E4
      Apolipoprotein C-III$_2$
    Familial lipoprotein lipase deficiency (during pregnancy)
    Familial combined hyperlipidemia (rarely)
  Secondary
    Diabetes mellitus
    Congenital lipodystrophy
    Obesity
    Oral contraceptives
    Alcohol
    Uremia
    Nephrotic syndrome
    Dysglobulinemias
    Hypothyroidism
    High-dose glucocorticoids
    Glycogen storage disease

References
1. Schaefer EJ, Levy RI: Pathogenesis and Management of Lipoprotein Disorders. *N Engl J Med* 312:1300, 1985.
2. Bierman EL, Glomset JA: Disorders of Lipid Metabolism. In general reference 9, p 1120.

4-L. Goiter (Including Nodules)

Diffuse Goiter
Euthyroid or hypothyroid
  Thyroiditis
    Hashimoto's thyroiditis
    Subacute (De Quervain's, granulomatous) thyroiditis
    Painless (silent) thyroiditis
    Acute (suppurative) thyroiditis
    Riedel's struma
  Defects in hormone synthesis (dyshormonogenesis)
  Iodine deficiency
  Ingestion of goitrogens
    Drugs
      Topical resorcinol
      Technetium perchlorate
      Thiocyanate
      Antithyroid agents
        Propylthiouracil
        Methimazole
        Carbimazole
      Sulfonamides
      p-Aminosalicylic acid
      Amphenone
      Phenylbutazone
      Iodides
      Lithium carbonate
      Cobalt
    Brassica genus (cabbage, turnips, brussel sprouts, rutabagas)
    Cassava
    Soybean milk/soybean flour
Hyperthyroid
  Graves' disease
  Subacute thyroiditis
  Painless (silent) thyroiditis
  "Hashitoxicosis"

Inappropriate thyroid-stimulating hormone (TSH) secre-
tion (rare)
Ectopic
Pituitary
With tumor
Without tumor

Multinodular Goiter
Nodular hyperplasia
Multiple adenomas

Solitary Nodule
Colloid nodule
Benign adenoma
Functional
Nonfunctional
Malignancy
Papillary carcinoma
Mixed papillary-follicular carcinoma
Follicular carcinoma
Lymphoma
Medullary carcinoma
Anaplastic carcinoma
Metastases to the thyroid
Thyroiditis
Hashimoto's thyroiditis
Subacute thyroiditis
Acute (suppurative) thyroiditis
Riedel's struma
Miscellaneous
Hematoma
Thyroid lobulation
Granulomatous disease
Clinically inapparent multinodular goiter
Nonthyroid adjacent mass (e.g., thyroglossal duct cyst)

Reference
1. Burrow GN: The Thyroid: Nodule and Neoplasia. In general reference 8, p 474.

4-M. Thyrotoxicosis

Thyrotoxicosis with hyperthyroidism (high or normal radio-
  active iodine uptake)
  Intrinsic thyroid autonomy
    Toxic adenoma
    Toxic multinodular goiter
  Abnormal thyroid stimulator
    Graves' disease
    Tumors secreting excessive human chorionic gonado-
      tropin (HCG)
      Choriocarcinoma
      Hydatidiform mole
      Embryonal cell carcinoma of testis
    Hashitoxicosis
  Inappropriate thyroid-stimulating hormone (TSH) secre-
    tion
    Pituitary adenoma
    Selective pituitary resistance to thyroid hormone
Thyrotoxicosis without hyperthyroidism (low radioactive io-
  dine uptake)
  Inflammatory diseases
    Subacute thyroiditis
    Painless ("silent") thyroiditis
  Extrathyroidal source of hormone
    Hormone ingestion (iatrogenic or factitious)
    Ectopic thyroid tissue
      Metastatic differentiated thyroid cancer
      Struma ovarii
Hyperthyroidism with low radioactive iodine uptake
  Iodine-induced thyrotoxicosis (Jod-Basedow)

Reference

1. Ingbar SH: Classification of the Causes of Thyrotoxicosis. In Ingbar SH, Braverman LE (eds): *Werner's The
  Thyroid.* Philadelphia: Lippincott, 1986, p 809.

4-N. Hypothyroidism

Primary hypothyroidism
  Thyroid agenesis
  Destruction of gland
    Surgical removal
    Radioactive iodine therapy
    External irradiation for nonthyroid malignancies
    Autoimmune disease
      Hashimoto's thyroiditis
    Replacement of thyroid tissue
      Thyroid cancer
      Cystinosis
      Metastatic nonthyroid cancer
      Lymphoma
      Sarcoidosis and other granulomatous diseases
      Amyloidosis
      Hemochromatosis
    Pan-thyroiditis
      Acute thyroiditis
      Painless thyroiditis
      Subacute thyroiditis
  Idiopathic atrophy (?autoimmune)
  Inhibition of thyroid hormone synthesis
    Iodine deficiency
    Inherited enzyme defects
    Drugs and goitrogens
      Propylthiouracil
      Methimazole
      Amiodarone
      Lithium
      Para-aminosalicylic acid
      Phenylbutazone
      Resorcinol
      Excess iodine in susceptible patients
      Cruciferous plants
      Cassava
      Cobalt
  Transient
    After surgery or radioactive iodine
    Postpartum
    In course of thyroiditis
  Peripheral resistance to thyroid hormone
Secondary (pituitary) or tertiary (hypothalamic)—see 4-P

References
1. Hoffenberg R: Primary Hypothyroidism. In Ingbar SH, Braverman LE (eds): *Werner's The Thyroid.* Philadelphia: Lippincott, 1986, p 1256.
2. Ingbar SH: The Thyroid Gland. In general reference 9, p 784.
3. Cassidy CE, Eddy RC: Hypothyroidism in Patients with Goiter. *Metabolism* 19:751, 1970.

4-O. Serum Thyroxine

Elevated
    Thyrotoxicosis (see 4-M)
    Therapy with D-thyroxine
    Elevated levels of serum thyroid-binding proteins
        Estrogens (endogenous or exogenous)
            Pregnancy
            Estrogen-containing medications (including oral contraceptives)
            Estrogen-secreting tumors
        Biliary cirrhosis
        Infections and chronic active hepatitis
        Neonatal state
        Perphenazine
        Genetically increased thyroxine-binding globulin
        Familial dysalbuminemic hyperthyroxinemia
        Acute intermittent porphyria
    Endogenous anti-T_4 antibodies
    Peripheral resistance to thyroid hormone
Decreased
    Hypothyroidism (primary or secondary) (see 4-N)
    Decreased levels of serum thyroid-binding proteins
        Protein loss (e.g., nephrotic syndrome)
        Severe systemic illness
        Genetically decreased thyroxine-binding globulin
        Androgens and anabolic steroids
        Chronic liver disease
        Acromegaly
        Glucocorticoid excess

Drugs
    Phenytoin
    Salicylates
    Therapy with T_3 alone

References

1. Wallach J: *Interpretation of Diagnostic Tests* (4th ed). Boston: Little, Brown, 1986, pp 80–82.
2. Larsen PR: Thyroid Hormone Concentrations. In Ingbar SH, Braverman LE: *Werner's The Thyroid*. Philadelphia: Lippincott, 1986, p 494.
3. Ingbar SH: The Thyroid Gland. In general reference 9, p 696.
4. Spaulding SW, Utiger RD: The Thyroid: Physiology, Hyperthyroidism, Hypothyroidism, and the Painful Thyroid. In general reference 8, p 405.

4-P. Pituitary/Hypothalamic Lesions

Invasive
    Craniopharyngioma
    Pituitary adenoma
    Meningioma
    Cyst
    Aneurysm
    Metastatic tumor
    Optic glioma
    Hamartoma
    Teratoma
    Ectopic pinealoma
    Leukemia
    Lymphoma
    Chordoma
Ischemic
    Sheehan's syndrome
    Diabetes mellitus
    Sickle cell anemia
    Collagen vascular disease
    Temporal arteritis
Infiltrative
    Hemochromatosis
    Sarcoidosis
    Amyloidosis
    Histiocytosis

Wegener's granulomatosis
Tay-Sachs disease
Injury
  Basilar skull fracture
Infectious
  Tuberculosis
  Meningitis
  Leukemia
  Fungal infections
  Encephalitis
  Syphilis
  Brucellosis
Immunologic
  Lymphocytic hypophysitis
Iatrogenic
  Surgery
  Radiation therapy
Idiopathic
Isolated
  Isolated growth hormone deficiency
  Isolated vasopressin deficiency
  Isolated adrenocorticotropic hormone (ACTH) deficiency
  Isolated thyroid-stimulating hormone (TSH) deficiency
  Isolated prolactin deficiency
  Kallmann's syndrome (hypothalamic hypogonadotropic
    hypogonadism)

References

1. Daughaday W: The Anterior Pituitary. In general reference 9, p 589.
2. Findling JW, Tyrrell JB: Anterior Pituitary and Somatomedins: I. Anterior Pituitary. In Greenspan FS, Forrham PH (Eds): *Basic and Clinical Endocrinology.* East Norwalk: Appleton-Century-Crofts, 1986, p 70.

5 EYE

5-A. Eye Pain

Foreign-Body Sensation
Foreign body on cornea, conjunctiva, or eyelid
Ingrown lashes, entropion
Corneal inflammation, abrasion, blebs, dystrophies

Burning Pain
Refractive error, uncorrected
Exposure to irritants (e.g., wind, dust, cosmetics)
Conjunctivitis
Insufficient secretions (including Sjögren's syndrome)
Corneal inflammation (keratitis)
    Infection
    Allergic blepharitis
    Trauma
    X-rays, ultraviolet light
    Associated with skin disease (e.g., psoriasis, erythema
      multiforme)

Aching, Boring Pain
Uveitis
Orbital periostitis, abscess
Herpes zoster infection

Retrobulbar neuritis
Tic douloureux
Aneurysm (e.g., circle of Willis)
Orbital neoplasm (primary or metastatic)

Tenderness, Pain upon Pressure
Lid inflammation
Dacryocystitis, dacryoadenitis (inflammation of lacrimal sac
    or gland)
Corneal foreign body, abrasion, ulcer
Conjunctivitis
Scleritis, episcleritis
Iritis, iridocyclitis
Orbital cellulitis, periostitis, or abscess
Glaucoma
Sinusitis
Fever
Headache

Reference
1. General reference 11, p 159.

5-B. Red Eye

Conjunctivitis
  Infection
    Bacterial
    Viral
    Chlamydial
    Spirochetal
    Fungal
  Drugs, especially:
    Local anesthetics
    Antibiotics (e.g., neomycin, sulfonamides, chloram-
      phenicol, tetracycline, erythromycin)
    Mydriatic and miotic drugs (e.g, atropine)
  Contact allergy (e.g., drugs, cosmetics)
  Vernal conjunctivitis
Ciliary injection
  Iritis, iridocyclitis (see 5-H)
  Acute narrow-angle glaucoma
  Corneal foreign body, abrasion, or ulceration
Chorioretinitis

Scleritis
Subconjunctival hemorrhage (traumatic or spontaneous)

Reference
1. General reference 11, p 359.

5-C. Loss or Impairment of Vision

Cornea
Corneal edema
Keratitis
   Viral infection (especially herpes)
   Congenital syphilis
   Behçet's syndrome
   Reiter's syndrome
   Stevens-Johnson syndome
   Allergic reactions
   Drying of eyes secondary to coma
   Mucopolysaccharidoses
Corneal dystrophies
Keratoconus

Aqueous Humor
Glaucoma

Vitreous Humor
Opacification
Hemorrhage (e.g., associated with diabetes, trauma, sickle
    cell disease)

Uveal Tract
Inflammation (see 5-H)
Hemorrhagic disease
Tumor, primary or metastatic

Lens
Refractive errors
   Myopia, hyperopia, presbyopia, astigmatism
   Lens sclerosis
   Large changes in blood sugar (e.g., diabetes mellitus)
Opacification (cataract)
   Age
   Diabetes mellitus

    Radiation
    Drugs (e.g., steroids, chlorpromazine)
    Hypoparathyroidism
    Congenital or hereditary causes (e.g., myotonic dystrophy, Fabry's disease, congenital rubella)
Dislocation
    Marfan's syndrome
    Homocystinuria

Retina

Degeneration
    Congenital or hereditary diseases (e.g., retinitis pigmentosa, Laurence-Moon-Biedl syndrome, pseudoxanthoma elasticum)
    Macular degeneration (hereditary or senile)
    Paget's disease
    Acromegaly
    Hyperphosphatemia
Vascular lesions
    Central retinal vein occlusion
        External compression
        Degenerative venous disease
        Diabetes mellitus
        Leukemia
        Sickle cell disease
        Trauma
        Inflammation, infection
    Central retinal artery occlusion
        Thrombus
        Embolus
        Spasm
        Temporal arteritis
    Carotid or basilar artery embolus or thrombosis
    Hemorrhage, especially:
        Diabetes mellitus
        Hypertension
        Severe anemia (e.g., sickle cell, massive blood loss)
        Thrombotic thrombocytopenic purpura, disseminated intravascular coagulation
Toxins, especially:
    Methanol
    Quinine
    Carbon bisulfide
Detachment
Retinitis or chorioretinitis
    Toxoplasmosis
    Histoplasmosis

Sarcoidosis
Lupus erythematosus
Polyarteritis nodosa
Tuberculosis
Syphilis
Cytomegalovirus infection
Bacterial sepsis, endocarditis
Tumor

Central Nervous System
Optic nerve disease
  Optic neuritis, neuropathy, atrophy (see 5-E)
  Prolonged papilledema
  Optic nerve trauma
Optic chiasm lesion
  Tumor (especially pituitary tumor, meningioma, meta-
    static tumor)
  Sarcoidosis
  Aneurysm of circle of Willis
Cerebral lesion
  Calcarine tract (optic radiation)
  Parietal lobe(s)
  Temporal lobe(s)
  Occipital lobe(s)
  Cortical blindness
  Migraine (usually transient)
  Head injury
  Hysteria

References
1. General reference 10, p 143.
2. General reference 11, p 159.
3. General reference 22, p 182.

5-D. Exophthalmos

Pseudoexophthalmos
  Unilateral ocular enlargement (e.g., trauma, myopia,
    glaucoma)*
Lid retraction
Extraocular muscle paralysis secondary to surgery or nerve
    injury*
Graves' disease
Orbital inflammation*
  Acute
    Cellulitis
    Abscess
    Periostitis
    Cavernous sinus thrombosis
  Chronic granulomatous ("pseudotumor")
    Sarcoidosis
    Tuberculosis
    Syphilis
Trauma*
  Orbital hemorrhage, hematoma
  Orbital fracture with air leak from sinus
Orbital tumor*
  Meningioma
  Dermoid
  Hemangioma
  Neuroblastoma
  Neurofibroma
  Optic nerve glioma
  Lymphoma, leukemic infiltrates
  Metastatic carcinoma
  Lacrimal gland tumor
  Rhabdomyosarcoma
Reticuloendotheliosis (especially Hand-Schüller-Christian
    disease)
Paranasal sinus or nasopharyngeal tumor, infection, muco-
    cele
Orbital cyst*
Orbital varices* (especially associated with trauma, arterio-
    venous malformation, hemangioma)
Orbital aneurysm* (e.g., ophthalmic artery)
Congenital (e.g., genetic, racial)

References
1. General reference 11, p 3.
2. Grove AS: Evaluation of Exophthalmos. *N Engl J Med*
   292:1005, 1975.

*Usually unilateral.

5-E. Optic Nerve Atrophy

Ocular diseases causing retinal degeneration (e.g., retinitis
   pigmentosa, extensive chorioretinitis)
Optic neuritis (optic nerve inflammation)
   Demyelinating disease
      Multiple sclerosis
      Diffuse cerebral sclerosis
      Schilder's disease
      Acute disseminated encephalomyelitis
      Neuromyelitis optica (Devic's disease)
   Infection: intraocular (keratitis, chronic uveitis, endoph-
      thalmitis) or extraocular (orbital cellulitis, meningitis,
      encephalitis, brain abscess)
      Bacterial (e.g., *Haemophilus influenzae*)
      Spirochetal (e.g., syphilis)
      Mycobacterial (e.g., tuberculosis)
      Viral (e.g., herpes zoster, mumps, measles, rubella; or
         mumps, measles, or rubella vaccine)
      Fungal (e.g., cryptococcus)
      Protozoal/helminthic (e.g., toxoplasmosis, toxocariasis)
      Guillain-Barré syndrome
Optic neuropathy
   Ischemic disease
      Arteriosclerosis, accelerated hypertension
      Collagen-vascular disease (e.g., lupus erythematosus,
         temporal arteritis, Behçet's syndrome, polyarteritis
         nodosa, Buerger's disease)
      Glaucoma
      Diabetes mellitus
      Sarcoidosis
      Hyperthyroidism
      Sickle cell disease
      Severe anemia
      Polycythemia vera
      Orbital radiation

Drugs, toxins
    Methanol
    Tobacco and/or alcohol
    Chloroquine
    Lead
    Arsenic
    Quinine
    Thallium
    Ethambutol
    Isoniazid
    Ergot
    Disulfiram
    Chloramphenicol
Nutritional deprivation (especially alcoholism, pellagra, beriberi, pernicious anemia)
Optic nerve trauma
Optic nerve tumor (e.g., optic nerve glioma, meningioma, metastatic carcinoma)
Prolonged papilledema (see 5-F)
Intracranial lesions affecting visual pathways (with or without papilledema)
Congenital and hereditary diseases (e.g., leukodystrophies, optic nerve hypoplasia)

References

1. General reference 22, p 182.
2. General reference 10, p 353.
3. Levine RA, Rosenberg MA, Rabb MF: The Optic Nerve. In Peyman, GA, Sanders DR, Goldberg MF (Eds): *Principles and Practice of Ophthalmology.* Philadelphia: Saunders, 1980, p 2091.

5-F. Papilledema*

Pseudotumor cerebri
Intracranial tumor (especially subtentorial)
    Meningioma
    Metastatic tumor
    Hodgkin's disease
    Optic nerve tumor
    Leukemia with optic nerve infiltrates
Infection (meningitis, encephalitis, brain abscess), especially:
    Bacterial
    Viral
    Tuberculous
    Syphilitic
    Fungal (especially cryptococcal)
Subarachnoid hemorrhage
Intracranial trauma (e.g., subdural or epidural hematoma, intracranial hemorrhage)
Vascular disease (involving retinal vessels)
    Hypertensive encephalopathy
    Collagen-vascular disease (especially lupus erythematosus)
    Granulomatous angiitis, other arteritides
    Central retinal vein occlusion
    Cavernous sinus thrombosis
Drugs and toxins
    Methanol
    Vitamin A
    Lead
    Arsenic
    Lithium
    Thallium
    Cisplatin
    Tetracycline
    Corticosteroids
    Progestins
    Nalidixic acid
Metabolic diseases
    Diabetes mellitus
    Adrenal insufficiency
    Hyperthyroidism
    Hypoparathyroidism
Sarcoidosis
Respiratory insufficiency with carbon dioxide retention

Congenital and developmental malformation (especially
  congenital hydrocephalus, craniosynostosis, Arnold-
  Chiari malformation, aqueductal stenosis)

***Optic Disk Blurring and/or Edema Without
Increased Intracranial Pressure***
Hyperopia
Medullated nerve fibers
Disk drusen
Orbital lesions (e.g., orbital hemangioma, perioptic menin-
  gioma)
Ocular hypotony (e.g., traumatic or surgical)
Ocular inflammatory disorders, especially:
  Uveitis (see 5-H)
  Optic neuritis (see 5-E)
  Papillophlebitis

References
1. General reference 10, p 353.
2. General reference 11, p 480.
3. Levine RA, Rosenberg MA, Rabb MF: The Optic Nerve.
   In Peyman GA, Sanders DR, Goldberg MF (Eds): *Principles and Practice of Ophthalmology.* Philadelphia:
   Saunders, 1980, p 2105.

---

*Optic disk swelling associated with increased intracranial pressure.

5-G. Pupillary Abnormalities

Miosis
Aging
Drugs (especially pilocarpine, morphine, physostigmine)
Corneal or conjunctival irritation
Iritis
Posterior synechiae (postinflammatory)
Pontine lesions
Meningitis, encephalitis
Cavernous sinus thrombosis
Neurosyphilis (Argyll Robertson pupil)
Congenital absence of dilator pupillae muscle

Mydriasis
Drugs, especially:
  Atropine
  Phenylephrine
  Isoproterenol
  Epinephrine
  Cocaine
Angle-closure glaucoma
Coma, especially due to:
  Alcohol intoxication
  Diabetes mellitus
  Uremia
  Postepilepsy
  Meningitis
  Midbrain lesions
Optic neuropathy or atrophy (see 5-E)
Intracranial neoplasm or aneurysm
Ocular trauma (especially with tear of iris sphincter muscle)
Orbital or cranial trauma
Orbital or choroidal tumor

Anisocoria
Local causes
  Mydriatic or miotic drugs
  Injury to iris (d)*
  Inflammation
    Keratitis (c)
    Iridocyclitis (d or c)
    Posterior synechiae (c)
  Angle-closure glaucoma (d)
  Ischemia of anterior ocular segment (e.g., resulting from
      internal carotid artery insufficiency) (d)
  Disease of iris (e.g., aniridia) (d)

Unilateral blindness resulting from optic or retinal
    causes (d)
Prosthetic eye
Sphincter pupillae muscle paralysis (d)
  Intracranial infection, especially:
    Syphilis
    Herpes zoster
    Tuberculosis
    Encephalitis, meningitis
    Botulism
    Diphtheria
  Intracranial neoplasm
  Cerebral aneurysm
  Cavernous sinus thrombosis
  Subdural, extradural hemorrhage
  Degenerative nervous system disease
  Toxic polyneuritis (especially alcohol, lead, arsenic)
  Diabetes mellitus
Dilator pupillae muscle paralysis (c) (see Horner's Syn-
    drome below)
Others
  Tabes dorsalis (c)
  Midbrain lesion (d)
  Adie's syndrome (d)

Horner's Syndrome
Peripheral causes; compression of, or injury to, cervical
    nerve roots, ganglia, or efferent sympathetic fibers
  Mediastinal tumor (especially bronchogenic carcinoma,
      metastatic tumor, Hodgkin's disease)
  Thyroid adenoma
  Neurofibromatosis
  Trauma (surgical or accidental)
  Internal carotid artery aneurysm
Central nervous system causes
  Posterior inferior cerebellar artery occlusion
  Multiple sclerosis
  Syringomyelia
  Brainstem or cervical cord tumor
  Spinal cord trauma
Congenital

Reference
1. General reference 10, p 274.

---

*"d" indicates the affected pupil is dilated; "c" indicates the affected
pupil is constricted.

5-H. Uveitis

Infection (local inflammation of orbit, cornea, conjunctiva; meningitis)
    Bacterial, especially:
        Staphylococcus aureus
        Proteus species
        Pseudomonas aeruginosa
        Bacillus subtilis
        Coliforms
        Neisseria gonorrhoeae
    Mycobacterial
        Tuberculosis
        Leprosy
    Spirochetal (syphilis)
    Viral, especially:
        Herpes simplex, herpes zoster
        Cytomegalovirus
        Variola
        Vaccinia
        Mononucleosis
        Lymphogranuloma venereum
    Rickettsial (typhus)
    Fungal (especially histoplasmosis)
    Protozoan, especially:
        Toxoplasmosis
        Amebic dysentery
        Malaria
        Sleeping sickness
Hypersensitivity reaction (especially air-borne allergens, foods, protein antigens)
Irritant or toxic gases
Trauma (especially sympathetic ophthalmia [following globe perforation], following lens rupture, retained foreign body)
Systemic disease
    Collagen-vascular disease
        Systemic lupus erythematosus
        Ankylosing spondylitis
        Juvenile rheumatoid arthritis
        Reiter's syndrome
        Behçet's syndrome
        Polyarteritis nodosa
        Wegener's granulomatosis
    Sarcoidosis
    Diabetes mellitus

Lens disease
   Hypermature cataract
   Retention of lens material after lens extraction
   Endophthalmitis phacoanaphylactica
Blindness with degenerative changes
Pars planitis
Necrosis of intraocular tumor
Idiopathic

References
1. General reference 10, p 283.
2. General reference 11, p 359.

6 GASTRO-INTESTINAL AND HEPATIC SYSTEMS

6-A. Nausea and Vomiting*

Gastrointestinal Disorders
Obstructive vomiting
  Any cause of bowel obstruction (see 6-I)
Nonobstructive vomiting
  Gastroenteritis
  Peptic ulcer disease
  Gastritis
  Pancreatitis
  Cholecystitis
  Gastroesophageal reflux
  Hepatitis
  Choledocholithiasis
  Biliary stricture
  Peritonitis
  Appendicitis
  Postvagotomy syndrome
  Diabetic gastroparesis
  Superior mesenteric artery (SMA) syndrome
  Prior gastrointestinal surgery
  Carcinoma: stomach, small intestine, pancreas, biliary
      tract
  Inflammatory bowel disease

Ischemic bowel disease
Idiopathic intestinal pseudoobstruction
Food poisoning
Eosinophilic gastroenteritis

Systemic Disorders
Acute infections (especially in children)
Reye's syndrome
Severe pain
Acute myocardial infarction
Congestive heart failure
Radiation sickness
Scleroderma
Amyloidosis
Acquired immunodeficiency syndrome (AIDS)

Central Nervous System Disorders
Intracranial hypertension
   Trauma
   Neoplasm
   Meningitis, encephalitis
   Hydrocephalus
Vestibular or middle ear disease
   Motion sickness
   Menière's disease
   Eighth nerve tumor
   Infection
Eye disorders
   Glaucoma
   Refractive error
Migraine headache
Autonomic epilepsy

Endocrine and Metabolic Disorders
Diabetic ketoacidosis
Metabolic acidosis from other causes
Uremia
Hypercalcemia
Hyponatremia
Hypothyroidism
Adrenal insufficiency
Hyperthyroidism
Hyperparathyroidism

Genitourinary Disorders
Pyelonephritis
Obstructive uropathy
Renal calculi

Salpingitis
Endometritis, parametritis

Drugs and Poisons
Chemotherapy
Alcohol
Anticholinergic drugs
Digitalis
Aminophylline
Colchicine
Morphine and derivatives
Ergot alkaloids
Antiarrhythmic drugs
Estrogens, oral contraceptives
Carbon monoxide
Carbon tetrachloride
Heavy metals (e.g., arsenic, mercury)

Miscellaneous
Pregnancy
   Hyperemesis gravidarum
Psychogenic
   Bulimia
   Anorexia nervosa
   Rumination
Alcohol, drug withdrawal

Reference
1. Feldman M: Nausea and Vomiting. In general reference 12, p 160.

*The causes of nausea and vomiting are innumerable. This list is not intended to include them all. The important categories of disorders with vomiting as a major symptom are listed, and several examples of each are given.

6-B. Dysphagia, Odynophagia

Oropharyngeal Causes
Painful swallowing
  Pharyngitis
  Herpes stomatitis
  Monilial stomatitis
  Mumps
  Vincent's angina
  Abscess
    Retropharyngeal
    Peritonsillar
  Malignancy
  Acute thyroiditis
Hypertonic cricopharyngeus muscle
Zenker's diverticulum
Pharyngeal paralysis
  Poliomyelitis
  Syringomyelia
  Cerebrovascular accident
  Amyotrophic lateral sclerosis
  Multiple sclerosis
  Glossopharyngeal neuritis
Pharyngeal muscle weakness
  Myasthenia gravis
  Myotonic dystrophy
  Restricted muscular dystrophy
    Oculopharyngeal
    Laryngeal esophageal
  Amyloidosis
  Scleroderma
  Dermatomyositis
Fixation of larynx
  Laryngeal neoplasm
  Scarring (e.g., secondary to tuberculosis)
Congenital abnormalities

Esophageal Causes
Motility disorders
  Achalasia
  Chagas' disease
  Scleroderma
  Diffuse esophageal spasm
  Diabetic neuropathy
  "Nutcracker" esophagus
  Presbyesophagus

Chronic idiopathic intestinal pseudoobstruction
Nonspecific esophageal dysmotility
Luminal narrowing
  Esophageal
    Reflux esophagitis
    Peptic stricture
    Carcinoma
    Esophageal web (Plummer-Vinson syndrome)
    Traumatic, corrosive stricture
    Contractile (Schatzki) ring
    Traction diverticulum
    Benign tumors
    Epiphrenic diverticulum
    Paraesophageal hernia
    Carcinoma of gastric cardia
  Extraesophageal, intrathoracic
    Lymph node enlargement (e.g., tuberculosis, malig-
       nancy)
    Thyromegaly (benign, malignant)
    Mediastinal disease
      Malignancy
      Tuberculosis
      Other inflammatory lesions
    Pulmonary abscess
    Empyema
    Pericardial effusion
    Vascular lesions
      Aortic aneurysm
      Anomalous right subclavian artery

References
1. Pope CE: Heartburn, Dysphagia, and Chest Pain of
   Esophageal Origin. In general reference 12, p 145.
2. Pope CE: The Esophagus. In general reference 12,
   p 407.
3. Eastwood GL: Esophageal Disorders. In general reference 13, p 3.

6-C. Abdominal Pain*

Abdominal Disorders
Intraperitoneal
  Inflammatory disorders
    Peritoneum
      Peritonitis (chemical or bacterial) (see 6-J)
      Subdiaphragmatic abscess
    Hollow viscera
      Gastroenteritis
      Appendicitis
      Cholecystitis
      Peptic ulcer disease
      Gastritis
      Duodenitis
      Crohn's disease
      Colitis
      Diverticulitis
    Solid viscera
      Pancreatitis (see 6-K)
      Hepatitis (see 6-O)
      Abscess (especially hepatic, splenic, pancreatic)
    Pelvic viscera
      Pelvic inflammatory disease
      Tuboovarian disease
      Mittelschmerz
      Endometritis
      Endometriosis
      Salpingitis
    Mesentery
      Mesenteric lymphadenitis
  Mechanical disorders
    Hollow viscera
      Intestinal obstruction
      Intussusception
      Biliary tract obstruction
    Solid viscera
      Acute capsular distension
        Acute splenomegaly
        Acute hepatomegaly (especially hepatitis, hepatic
          congestion, Budd-Chiari syndrome)
    Pelvic viscera
      Ovarian cyst/torsion
      Ectopic pregnancy
    Mesentery
      Omental torsion

Malignancy
   Pancreatic
   Gastric
   Hepatic, primary or metastatic
   Colonic
   Small intestinal
   Ovarian
   Uterine
Vascular disorders
   Intraabdominal bleeding
   Ischemia
      Mesenteric artery insufficiency or thrombosis
      Infarction (especially liver, spleen)
      Omental ischemia
Extraperitoneal
  Pyelonephritis
  Ureteral obstruction (especially stones, tumor)
  Aortic aneurysm
    Rupture
    Dissection
    Expansion
  Perinephric abscess
  Psoas abscess
  Prostatitis
  Seminal vesiculitis
  Epididymitis

Extraabdominal Disorders
Thoracic
  Lung
    Pneumonia
    Pulmonary infarction
    Pneumothorax
    Empyema
    Pleuritis
  Heart
    Myocardial ischemia or infarction
    Pericarditis
    Myocarditis, endocarditis
  Esophagus
    Esophagitis
    Esophageal spasm
    Esophageal rupture
Neurologic
  Radiculitis
    Herpes zoster
    Degenerative arthritis

    Herniated intervertebral disk
    Tumor
  Causalgia
  Tabes dorsalis
Hematologic
  Leukemia
  Lymphoma
  Sickle cell crisis
Abdominal wall
  Contusion
  Hematoma
Toxins
  Insect bites (especially from black widow spiders)
  Snake venom
Metabolic disorders
  Uremia
  Diabetes (especially ketoacidosis)
  Addisonian crisis
  Porphyria
  Lead colic
  Hyperlipidemia
  Hereditary angioneurotic edema
Psychiatric disorders
  Depression
  Hysteria
  Schizophrenia
  Factitious abdominal pain
Other
  Acute glaucoma

Reference

1. Way LW: Abdominal Pain. In general reference 12, p 207.

*See also 6-D.

6-D. Characteristic Location of Abdominal Pain Associated with Various Diseases*

Diffuse
Gastroenteritis
Peritonitis
Pancreatitis
Leukemia
Sickle cell crisis
Early appendicitis (may be periumbilical)
Mesenteric adenitis
Mesenteric thrombosis
Abdominal aortic aneurysm
Intussusception
Colitis
Intestinal obstruction
Inflammatory bowel disease
Metabolic, toxic, bacterial causes

Epigastric
Peptic ulcer disease
Pancreatitis
Gastritis
Cholecystitis
Reflux esophagitis
Myocardial ischemia
Pericarditis
Abdominal wall hematoma

Right Upper Quadrant
Cholecystitis
Choledocholithiasis
Hepatitis
Hepatic metastases
Hepatic abscess
Hepatocellular carcinoma
Hepatomegaly resulting from congestive heart failure
Budd-Chiari syndrome (hepatic vein obstruction)
Peptic ulcer
Pancreatitis
Retrocecal appendicitis
Renal pain
Herpes zoster
Myocardial ischemia
Pericarditis

Pneumonia
Empyema
Pulmonary infarction
Pleuritis

Left Upper Quadrant
Gastritis
Peptic ulcer disease
Pancreatitis
Splenic
   Enlargement, rupture
   Infarction, aneurysm
Renal pain
Herpes zoster
Myocardial ischemia
Pericarditis
Pneumonia
Empyema
Pulmonary infarction
Pleuritis

Right Lower Quadrant
Appendicitis
Intestinal obstruction
Crohn's disease
Diverticulitis
Cholecystitis
Perforated ulcer
Leaking aortic aneurysm
Abdominal wall hematoma
Ectopic pregnancy
Ovarian cyst or torsion
Salpingitis
Mittelschmerz
Endometriosis
Ureteral colic
Renal pain
Seminal vesiculitis
Psoas abscess

Left Lower Quadrant
Diverticulitis
Intestinal obstruction
Colon cancer
Appendicitis
Gastritis
Leaking aortic aneurysm
Inflammatory bowel disease

Abdominal wall hematoma
Splenic distention
Ectopic pregnancy
Mittelschmerz
Ovarian cyst or torsion
Salpingitis
Endometriosis
Ureteral colic
Renal pain
Seminal vesiculitis
Psoas abscess

*Modified from Schwartz SI, Storer EH: Manifestations of Gastrointestinal Disease. In Schwartz SI, Shires GT, Spencer FC, Storer EH (Eds): *Principles of Surgery* (4th ed). New York: McGraw-Hill, 1984, p 1026. Copyright 1984 by McGraw-Hill Book Company.

6-E. Constipation

Simple Constipation
Low-residue diet
Chronic laxative and/or enema abuse
Muscular weakness

Gastrointestinal Disorders
Colonic, extraluminal obstruction
   Tumors
   Chronic volvulus
   Hernias
   Rectal prolapse
   Ascites
   Pregnancy
   Adhesions
Colonic, luminal disorders
   Tumors (benign, malignant)
   Fecal impaction
   Diverticulitis
   Strictures
      Chronic ulcerative colitis
      Recurrent diverticulitis
      Carcinoma
      Chronic amebiasis
      Lymphogranuloma venereum
      Syphilis
      Tuberculosis

    Ischemic colitis
    Endometriosis
    Postsurgical
  Intussusception
Anorectal disorders
  Proctitis (especially ulcerative)
  Hemorrhoids
  Fissures and fistulas (e.g., Crohn's disease)
  Perianal abscess
  Rectal prolapse
  Stenosis
    Neoplastic
    Inflammatory (especially lymphogranuloma venereum)
    Postsurgical
  Puborectalis syndrome
Abnormalities of muscle function
  Irritable bowel syndrome
  Diverticular disease
  Myotonic dystrophy
  Scleroderma
  Dermatomyositis

Neuromuscular Disorders

Spinal cord disorders (especially trauma, multiple sclerosis,
    cauda equina tumor)
Diabetic autonomic neuropathy
Muscular abnormality

Peripheral Nerve Disorders

Hirschsprung's disease
von Recklinghausen's disease
Chagas' disease
Multiple endocrine neoplasia, type IIB
Colonic pseudoobstruction

Neurologic and Psychiatric Disorders

Psychotic depression
Senility
Cerebrovascular accident
Parkinson's disease
Central nervous system tumor

Endocrine and Metabolic Disorders

Diabetes (with neuropathy)
Hypothyroidism
Hyperparathyroidism
Other hypercalcemic states
Pheochromocytoma

Hypokalemia
Panhypopituitarism
Lead poisoning
Uremia
Porphyria
Amyloidosis

Drugs
Antacids
  Calcium carbonate
  Aluminum hydroxide
Opiates
Anticholinergics
Anticonvulsants
Tricyclic antidepressants
Ganglionic blockers
Phenothiazines
Diuretics
Ferrous sulfate
Antihypertensives
Barium sulfate
Bismuth compounds
Ion-exchange resins

Reference
1. DeVroede G: Constipation: Mechanism and Management. In general reference 12, p 288.

6-F. Diarrhea

Acute Diarrhea
Infectious
  Viral gastroenteritis
  Bacterial
    Invasive (e.g., *Shigella, Salmonella, Campylobacter,*
       invasive *Escherichia coli, Yersinia*)
    Toxigenic (e.g., *Staphylococcus, E. coli, Clostridia,*
       Vibrio species)
  Protozoal (e.g., amebiasis, giardiasis)
Acquired immunodeficiency syndrome (AIDS)
Stress-induced
Traveler's diarrhea
Food allergy (rare)
Dietary indiscretion (e.g., prunes, unripe fruit, rhubarb)
Excessive alcohol ingestion
Gastrointestinal disorders
  Partial bowel obstruction
  Diverticulitis
  Appendicitis
  Ischemic bowel disease
  Pseudomembranous colitis
  Initial attack of ulcerative colitis or Crohn's disease
Systemic disorders
  Uremia
  Carcinoid syndrome
  Endocrine disorders
    Thyrotoxicosis
    Addisonian crisis
Poisoning
  Heavy metals (especially arsenic, cadmium, mercury)
  Mushrooms
Drugs
  Laxatives
  Broad-spectrum antibiotics
  Magnesium-containing antacids
  Lactulose
  Colchicine
  Digitalis
  Iron
  Guanethidine
  Methyldopa
  Hydralazine
  Quinidine
Acute exacerbation of chronic diarrhea

Chronic Diarrhea

Mucosal inflammation
  Ulcerative colitis, proctitis
  Crohn's disease
  Amebic colitis
  Radiation enterocolitis
  Ischemic colitis
  Pseudomembranous colitis
  Diverticulitis
  Parasitic infestation

Decreased solute absorption (osmotic diarrhea)
  Disaccharidase deficiency
  Monosaccharide malabsorption
  Postgastrectomy "dumping" syndrome
  Congenital chloridorrhea
  Malabsorption syndromes (see 6-G)
  Maldigestion syndromes (see 6-G)

Secretory diarrhea
  Zollinger-Ellison syndrome (gastrinoma)
  Pancreatic cholera (VIPoma)
  Carcinoid syndrome
  Medullary carcinoma of the thyroid
  Hydroxy fatty acid excretion
  Bile salt malabsorption
  Sympathetic tissue tumors (ganglioneuromas)
  Food allergy
  Villous adenoma
  Carotid body tumor

Motor disorders
  Irritable bowel syndrome
  Neoplasm (obstruction)
  Postvagotomy
  Postsurgical
  Gastrectomy
  Gastroenterostomy
  Pyloroplasty
  Gastroileal or gastrocolonic fistula

Miscellaneous

Eosinophilic gastroenteritis
Protein-losing enteropathy
Systemic diseases
  Endocrine disorders
    Addison's disease
    Hyperthyroidism
    Hypoparathyroidism
  Collagen-vascular disorders

    Systemic lupus erythematosus
    Scleroderma
    Polyarteritis nodosa
  Others
    Acquired immunodeficiency syndrome (AIDS)
    Uremia
    Neuropathic disorders (especially diabetes mellitus, amyloidosis, postvagotomy state)
    Cirrhosis
    Chronic cholecystitis
    Deficiency syndromes
      Pernicious anemia
      Pellagra
    Immunoglobulin deficiencies
Drugs (see also Acute Diarrhea above)
    Chronic opiate abuse

References

1. Krejs GJ: Diarrhea. In general reference 12, p 257.
2. Donowitz M: Pathophysiology of Diarrhea. In general reference 13, p 73.

6-G. Maldigestion, Malabsorption Syndromes

Maldigestion Syndromes

Pancreatic disorders
  Chronic pancreatitis
  Pancreatic resection
  Pancreatic carcinoma
  Cystic fibrosis
  Non-beta islet cell tumors
  Severe protein malnutrition
  Effect of vagotomy on pancreatic secretion
Hepatobiliary disease
  Extrahepatic biliary obstruction
  Chronic intrahepatic cholestasis (e.g., primary biliary cirrhosis)
  Severe hepatocellular injury
Impaired enzyme or bile salt function due to:
  Inadequate mixing (e.g., following gastrectomy, gastrojejunostomy, vagotomy, pyloroplasty, Billroth I or II)
  Acid pH in small bowel (e.g., Zollinger-Ellison syndrome)

Ileal resection
Severe diffuse ileal disease (e.g., Crohn's disease)

Malabsorption Syndromes
Mucosal cell abnormality
  Sprue
    Celiac
    Tropical
    Collagenous
  Whipple's disease
  Inflammatory diseases
    Crohn's disease
    Infectious enteritis
      Bacterial
      Tuberculous
      Parasitic (e.g., *Giardia, Coccidia*)
  Short-bowel syndrome
    Massive resection (especially for Crohn's disease)
    Enteroenteric fistulas
    Jejunoileal bypass surgery
    Gastroileal anastomosis (inadvertent)
  Bacterial overgrowth as a result of stasis
    Surgical blind loop
    Stricture, fistula
    Crohn's disease
    Small-bowel diverticula
    Hypomotility states
      Intestinal diabetic neuropathy
      Scleroderma
      Intestinal pseudoobstruction
  Disaccharidase deficiency
    Lactase
    Sucrase-isomaltase
  Others
    Ischemic bowel disease
    Radiation enteritis
    Nongranulomatous ulcerative jejunitis
    Abetalipoproteinemia
    Hypogammaglobulinemia
    Chloridorrhea, congenital or acquired
Infiltrative diseases
  Lymphoma
    Primary intestinal
    Extraintestinal
  Amyloidosis
  Eosinophilic gastroenteritis
  Mastocytosis
Intestinal congestion

Congestive heart failure
Constrictive pericarditis
Lymphatic obstruction
    Intestinal lymphangiectasia
    Tuberculosis
    Retroperitoneal malignancy

Systemic Disorders
Endocrine disorders
    Diabetes mellitus
    Hypoparathyroidism
    Hyperthyroidism
    Hypothyroidism
    Adrenal insufficiency
Protein malnutrition
Collagen-vascular disease
    Systemic lupus erythematosus
    Scleroderma
Dermatologic disorders
    Dermatitis herpetiformis
    Psoriasis
Food allergy
Others
    Pernicious anemia
    Carcinoid syndrome
    Iron deficiency
    Dysgammaglobulinemia, heavy-chain
    Genetic disorders of membrane transport (e.g., Hartnup
        disease)

Drugs
Cholestyramine
Colchicine
Broad-spectrum antibiotics (e.g., neomycin)
Cytotoxic drugs
Irritant laxatives
Phenindione

References
1. Gray GM: Maldigestion and Malabsorption: Clinical Manifestations and Specific Diagnosis. In general reference 12, p 228.
2. Symposium on Malabsorption. *Am J Med* 67:979, 1979.
3. Eastwood GL: Malabsorption Syndrome. In general reference 13, p 89.

6-H. Gastrointestinal Bleeding

Upper Gastrointestinal Bleeding
Acute (these account for > 90% of cases)
  Peptic ulcer disease
  Erosive gastritis
  Ruptured esophagogastric varices
  Mallory-Weiss tear
Chronic/occult sources
  Peptic ulcer disease
    Duodenal ulcer
    Gastric ulcer
    Stress ulcer
    Marginal/stomal ulcer
    Intestinal ulceration (e.g., associated with use of en-
      teric-coated potassium chloride)
  Erosive gastritis, duodenitis
    Peptic
    Alcohol
    Drug-induced
      Acetylsalicylic acid
      Nonsteroidal anti-inflammatory drugs (NSAID)
  Esophageal sources
    Gastroesophageal reflux
    Barrett's esophagitis
    Monilial esophagitis
    Herpetic esophagitis
    Esophageal rupture (Boerhaave syndrome)
  Neoplasms
    Carcinoma of esophagus, stomach, small intestine
    Polyps (primarily gastric)
    Leiomyoma
    Lymphoma
    Sarcoma
    Neurofibroma
    Carcinoid
    Hemangioma
    Plasmacytoma
  Ischemic bowel disease (especially mesenteric vascular
    occlusion)
  Bleeding disorders (e.g., anticoagulant therapy)
  Others
    Aortointestinal fistula
      Leaking aneurysm
      Aortic prosthesis
    Osler-Rendu-Weber syndrome
    Hereditary telangiectasis

Angiodysplasia
Uremia
Amyloidosis
Hemobilia
    Traumatic
    Ruptured hepatic artery aneurysm
Vasculitis (especially polyarteritis nodosa, systemic lupus erythematosus)
Blue rubber nevus bleb syndrome
Esophagogastric varices after partial sclerotherapy
Epistaxis with swallowed blood
Ehlers-Danlos syndrome
Pseudoxanthoma elasticum
Hemoptysis

Lower Gastrointestinal Bleeding
Acute (these account for > 90% of cases)
    Diverticulosis
    Ischemic colitis
    Angiodysplasia
    Colonic polyps
    Carcinoma
    Hemorrhoids
    Radiation colitis
Chronic/occult sources
    Anorectal lesions
        Hemorrhoids
        Anal fissures/fistulas
        Proctitis
        Trauma
    Colonic lesions
        Neoplasms
            Carcinoma of rectum, colon
            Polyps
                Tubular adenomas
                Villous adenomas
                Familial colonic polyposis
                Gardner's syndrome
                Peutz-Jeghers syndrome
                Juvenile polyposis
            Others
                Leiomyoma
                Sarcoma
                Lymphoma
                Neurofibroma
                Hemangioma
        Chronic inflammatory bowel disease
            Ulcerative colitis

Crohn's disease
Infectious colitis
  Bacterial (especially *Shigella, Salmonella,* pathogenic *Escherichia coli*)
  Mycobacterial (especially tuberculosis)
  Parasitic (especially amebiasis, schistosomiasis, whipworm)
  Spirochetal (especially syphilis)
  Viral
Ischemic colitis (e.g., mesenteric artery occlusion)
Pseudomembranous colitis
Radiation colitis
Diverticular disease
  Diverticulitis
  Meckel's diverticulum
Mechanical abnormalities
  Incarcerated hernia
  Volvulus
  Intussusception
  Foreign body
Systemic diseases
  Bleeding disorder (see 8-O)
  Uremia
  Amyloidosis
  Vasculitis
    Polyarteritis nodosa
    Systemic lupus erythematosus
    Henoch-Schönlein purpura
    Dermatomyositis
Others
  Aortointestinal fistula
  Arteriovenous malformation
  Osler-Rendu-Weber syndrome
  Submucosal vascular ectasia (angiodysplasia)
  Blue rubber nevus bleb syndrome
  Pseudoxanthoma elasticum
  Ehlers-Danlos syndrome
  Whipple's disease

References
1. Peterson WL: Gastrointestinal Bleeding. In general reference 12, p 177.
2. Eastwood GL: Gastrointestinal Bleeding. In general reference 13, p 216.

6-I. Abdominal Distention

Mechanical Bowel Obstruction
Extraluminal compression
  Adhesions
    Postsurgical
    Inflammatory
    Neoplastic
    Congenital
  Intraabdominal abscess
  Hematoma
  Neoplasm
  Pregnancy
  Annular pancreas
  Superior mesenteric artery (SMA) syndrome
Intraluminal obstruction
  Neoplasm
    Benign
    Malignant
  Inflammatory disorders (e.g., Crohn's disease, ulcerative
      colitis, diverticulitis)
  Trauma
  Foreign body
  Gallstones
  Parasites (especially *Ascaris*)
  Fecaliths
  Enteroliths
  Bezoars
  Food boluses
  Meconium
  Pneumatosis intestinalis
Intussusception
Volvulus
Hernias
Obstruction at surgical anastomosis
Congenital defect (e.g., Hirschsprung's disease)
Others
  Radiation stenosis
  Endometriosis

Adynamic Ileus, Nonmechanical Obstruction
Intraabdominal causes
  Peritoneal inflammation (see 6-J)
  Traumatic
    Postoperative
    Penetrating wounds
  Bacterial infections

Chemical irritants
  Blood
  Gastric contents (perforated ulcer)
  Bile
  Pancreatic enzymes (acute pancreatitis)
Vascular insufficiency
  Strangulation
    Intramural (distention resulting from mechanical
      ileus)
    Extramural (compression of mesenteric vessels)
  Mesenteric artery thrombosis or embolus
Retroperitoneal irritation
  Retroperitoneal hemorrhage
  Psoas abscess
  Pyelonephritis
  Renal colic
  Perinephric abscess
  Pancreatitis
  Pancreatic abscess
  Cancer
  Lymphoma
Extraabdominal causes
  Mechnical ventilation
  Toxic, metabolic
    Pneumonia
    Empyema
    Uremia
    Porphyria
    Severe systemic infection
    Heavy metal poisoning (e.g., lead)
  Traumatic
    Thoracic
    Retroperitoneal
    Intracranial
    Spinal
  Severe electrolyte imbalance (e.g., hypokalemia)
  Other
    Osteomyelitis of spine

Vascular Obstruction
Mesenteric artery thrombosis or embolus
Venous thrombosis

Idiopathic Intestinal Pseudoobstruction

Excessive Intraluminal Gas
Aerophagia
Increased intestinal gas production

Ascites (see 6-Q)

Reference
1. Jones RS: Intestinal Obstruction, Pseudo-obstruction, and Ileus. In general reference 12, p 308.

6-J. Peritonitis

Infections
  Bacterial
    Acute bacterial peritonitis
    Primary or spontaneous bacterial peritonitis (SBP), usually in cirrhotics with ascites
  Mycobacterial (primarily tuberculosis)
  Fungal (rare), especially:
    Candidiasis
    Histoplasmosis
    Cryptococcosis
    Coccidioidomycosis
  Parasitic (rare), especially:
    Schistosomiasis
    Ascariasis
    Enterobiasis
    Amebiasis
    Strongyloidiasis
Spontaneous perforation of viscus
  Peptic ulcer disease
  Appendicitis
  Gangrenous cholecystitis
  Diverticulitis
  Strangulated bowel
    Small-bowel adhesion
    Incarcerated hernia
    Volvulus
  Perforating carcinoma
  Ulcerative colitis (especially with toxic megacolon)
  Ischemic bowel
  Ingested foreign body
  Meckel's diverticulum
Ruptured visceral abscess or cyst, especially:
  Liver
  Kidney
  Spleen

Tuboovarian
Trauma, iatrogenic
  Penetrating wounds
  Surgical injury
  Instrumentation
    Sigmoidoscopy or colonoscopy
    Gastroscopy
    Abortion
    Paracentesis
Neoplasms
  Primary mesothelioma
  Secondary carcinomatosis
  Pseudomyxoma peritonei
Vasculitis
  Systemic lupus erythematosus
  Allergic vasculitis (Henoch-Schönlein purpura)
  Köhlmeier-Degos disease
Granulomatous peritonitis
  Parasitic infestations
  Sarcoidosis
  Tumors
  Crohn's disease
  Starch granules
Gynecologic disorders
  Endometriosis
  Teratoma
  Leiomyomatosis
  Dermoid cyst
  Melanosis
Chemical irritants
  Bile
  Blood
  Gastric juice
  Barium
  Enema or douche contents
Others
  Chronic peritoneal dialysis
  Eosinophilic peritonitis
  Chylous peritonitis (see 6-Q, under Chylous ascites)
  Whipple's disease
  Sclerosing peritonitis
  Peritoneal lymphangiectasis
  Peritoneal encapsulation
  Peritoneal loose bodies and peritoneal cysts
  Mesothelial hyperplasia and metaplasia
  Splenosis
  Familial paroxysmal polyserositis (familial Mediterranean fever)

Reference
1. Bender MD, Ockner RK: Diseases of the Peritoneum, Mesentery and Diaphragm. In general reference 12, p 1569.

6-K. Pancreatitis

Biliary tract disease
  Gallstone pancreatitis
  Choledocholithiasis
Alcoholic pancreatitis
  Acute
  Chronic recurrent (relapsing)
Idiopathic
Peptic ulcer disease (especially penetrating duodenal or gastric ulcer)
Trauma
  Blunt or penetrating
  Surgical
Duodenal disease
  Spasm of sphincter of Oddi
  Obstruction of sphincter of Oddi
    Fibrosis, stenosis
    Edema
    Tumor
  Crohn's disease
  Periampullary diverticulum
Neoplasm
  Head of pancreas
  Pancreatic carcinoma with duct obstruction
  Carcinoma of ampulla of Vater
  Metastatic carcinoma
Congenital pancreatic disorders
  Pancreas divisum
  Hereditary (familial) pancreatitis
Acquired pancreatic disorders
  Fibrosis
  Calculi
  Ductal strictures
  Pseudocyst
  Abscess
Metabolic disorders
  Hyperlipoproteinemia (types I, IV, and V)
  Hyperparathyroidism
  Other hypercalcemic states

Drugs
    Azathioprine
    Thiazide diuretics
    Ethacrynic acid
    Furosemide
    Tetracycline
    Salicylazosulfapyridine
    L-Asparaginase
    Oral contraceptives
    Corticosteroids
    Estrogens
Toxins
    Methyl alcohol
    Scorpion venom (Trinidad)
Infectious agents
    Mumps
    Coxsackie B infection
    Viral hepatitis
    Legionnaire's disease
    Campylobacter
    Mycoplasma
    Ascaris infestation
Vascular insufficiency or infarction
Miscellaneous
    Protein-calorie malnutrition
    Pregnancy
    Hypothermia
    Cardiopulmonary bypass surgery
    Hypotensive shock
    Endoscopic retrograde cholangiopancreatography
    Upper gastrointestinal endoscopy
    Posttransplantation
    Acquired immunodeficiency syndrome (AIDS)

References

1. Salt WB, Schenker S: Amylase—Its Clinical Significance: A Review of the Literature. *Medicine* 55:269, 1976.
2. The Pancreas. In general reference 12, p 1415.
3. Steinberg WM: Acute Pancreatitis. In general reference 13, p 233.

6-L. Hyperamylasemia Not Associated with Pancreatitis

Intraabdominal Disorders
Biliary tract disease, common duct stones
Perforated peptic ulcer not in contact with pancreas
Intestinal infarction
Intestinal obstruction
Intestinal perforation
Afferent loop syndrome
Ruptured ectopic pregnancy
Salpingitis
Dissecting aortic aneurysm
Peritonitis
Appendicitis

Salivary Gland Disorders
Parotitis (especially mumps)
Calculi
Radiation sialoadenitis
Maxillofacial surgery
Drugs
   Oxyphenbutazone
   Phenylbutazone

Miscellaneous
Chronic renal insufficiency
Salivary-type hyperamylasemia
Malignancy (especially lung)
Macroamylasemia
Cerebral trauma
Burns
Traumatic shock
Postoperative hyperamylasemia
Diabetic ketoacidosis
Renal transplantation
Pneumonia
Acquired bisalbuminemia
Prostatic disease
Pregnancy
Drugs
   Opiates

Reference
1. Salt WB, Schenker S: Amylase—Its Clinical Significance: A Review of the Literature. *Medicine* 55:269, 1976.

6-M. Hepatomegaly

Palpable Liver Without Hepatic Pathology
Normal variant
Thin or flaccid abdominal wall
Depressed right diaphragm (e.g., emphysema)
Subdiaphragmatic lesion (e.g., abscess)
Riedel's lobe

True Hepatic Enlargement
Inflammatory liver disease
  Hepatitis (see 6-O)
    Infectious
      Viral
      Schistosomiasis
      Other
    Alcoholic
    Other toxins
    Drug-induced
    Autoimmune
    Other
  Abscess
    Pyogenic
    Amebic
  Cholangitis
    Suppurative
    Sclerosing
  Pericholangitis (especially ulcerative colitis)
Chronic liver disease, cirrhosis (see 6-P)
  Alcoholic
  Posthepatitic
  Postnecrotic
  Metabolic disorders
  Other causes
Extrahepatic biliary obstruction
  Choledocholithiasis
  Biliary stricture
  Pancreatitis
  Carcinoma
    Bile ducts
    Head of pancreas
    Ampulla of Vater
  External compression
Hepatic congestion
  Congestive heart failure
  Constrictive pericarditis
  Budd-Chiari syndrome (hepatic outflow obstruction)

Thrombosis
Tumor
Infiltrative disorders, storage diseases
  Lipid accumulation
    Fatty liver
      Alcohol
      Diabetes mellitus
      Obesity
      Severe protein malnutrition
      Nonalcoholic steatonecrosis
      Jejunoileal bypass
      Parenteral hyperalimentation
      Corticosteroids, Cushing's syndrome
      Fatty liver of pregnancy
      Massive tetracycline therapy
      Toxins (e.g., carbon tetrachloride, DDT)
      Reye's syndrome
    Lipid storage disease (especially Gaucher's disease,
      Niemann-Pick disease)
  Glycogen accumulation
    Glycogen storage disease
    Diabetic glycogenosis
  Granulomatous infiltration (especially sarcoidosis, miliary
    tuberculosis, disseminated fungal diseases, some
    drug reactions)
  Myelo- and lymphoproliferative disorders
    Lymphoma
    Myeloid metaplasia
    Multiple myeloma
    Leukemia
  Amyloidosis
  Congenital hepatic fibrosis
  Hemochromatosis
  Wilson's disease
  Alpha$_1$-antitrypsin deficiency
  Hurler's syndrome
Neoplasms
  Primary
    Malignant
      Hepatocellular carcinoma
      Cholangiocarcinoma
      Angiosarcoma
    Benign
      Adenoma
      Hemangioma
      Focal nodular hyperplasia
  Metastatic
    Pancreas

Colon
Lung
Breast
Stomach
Kidney
Esophagus
Carcinoid
Cysts
  Congenital
    Solitary
    Polycystic
  Acquired (especially echinococcal)

References
1. Isselbacher KJ: Jaundice and Hepatomegaly. In general reference 12, p 183.
2. General reference 14.

6-N. Jaundice

Primarily Unconjugated Hyperbilirubinemia
Increased production
  Hemolysis, intravascular or extravascular (see 8-B)
  Ineffective erythropoiesis
  Hematomas, pulmonary embolus
Decreased hepatic uptake
  Gilbert's syndrome
  Drugs
    Flavaspidic acid
    Iodinated contrast agents
    Rifampin
  Posthepatitis
  Decreased cystolic binding proteins (e.g., newborn or premature infants)
  Portocaval shunt
  Prolonged fasting
Decreased glucuronyl transferase activity
  Crigler-Najjar syndrome, types I and II
  Gilbert's syndrome
  Physiologic jaundice of newborn
  Breast-milk jaundice
  Chronic persistent hepatitis
  Wilson's disease
  Noncirrhotic portal fibrosis

Primarily Conjugated Hyperbilirubinemia
Decreased liver excretion, intrahepatic
    Familial or hereditary disorders
        Dubin-Johnson syndrome
        Rotor syndrome
        Benign recurrent intrahepatic cholestasis
        Intrahepatic cholestasis of pregnancy
    Acquired disorders
        Hepatitis (see 6-O)
        Cirrhosis (see 6-P)
        Alcoholic liver disease
        Primary sclerosing cholangitis
        Pericholangitis
        Drugs and toxins, especially:
            Chlorpromazine
            Erythromycin estolate
            Isoniazid
            Halothane
    Others
        Hepatic malignancy, primary or metastatic
        Congestive heart failure
        Shock
        Sepsis
        Toxemia of pregnancy
        Hepatic trauma
        Sarcoidosis
        Amyloidosis
Extrahepatic biliary obstruction
    Congenital
        Bile duct atresia
        Idiopathic dilatation of common bile duct
        Cystic fibrosis
    Acquired
        Cholecystitis
        Common bile duct obstruction
            Choledocholithiasis
            Tumors (benign, malignant)
                Gallbladder
                Bile ducts
                Ampulla of Vater
                Pancreas
            External compression
            Strictures
                Common bile duct
                Sphincter of Oddi
            Pancreatitis
            Sclerosing cholangitis

References

1. Walkoff AW (Ed): Bilirubin Metabolism and Hyperbilirubinemia. *Semin Liver Dis,* Vol 3, No 1, 1983.
2. General reference 14.
3. Zawacki JK: Jaundice and Bilirubin Metabolism. In general reference 13, p 281.

6-O. Hepatitis, Abnormal "Liver Function Tests"

Most Common Etiologic Types (> 90% of cases)
Viral hepatitis (A and B)
Alcoholic hepatitis
Drug-induced hepatitis

Infection
Viral
    Hepatitis A
    Hepatitis B
    Non-A, non-B hepatitis
    Delta hepatitis
    Infectious mononucleosis (Epstein-Barr virus)
    Cytomegalovirus
    Varicella zoster
    Coxsackie
    Rubella
    Measles
    Herpes simplex
    Other
Bacterial (not necessarily hepatitis, per se)
    Pyogenic abscesses
        Numerous aerobic and anaerobic organisms
    Hepatic dysfunction in bacterial sepsis
        Escherichia coli
        Klebsiella pneumoniae
        Pseudomonas aeruginosa
        Proteus species
        Bacteroides species
        Staphylococcus aureus
        Aerobic and anaerobic streptococci
    Hepatic dysfunction in gram-positive infections
        Pneumococcal
        Streptococcal
        Staphylococcal

    Clostridia species
  Hepatic dysfunction in gram-negative infections
    E. coli
    Paracolon bacteria
    Pseudomonas aeruginosa
    Proteus
    Bacteroides
    Aerobacter
    Klebsiella
    Enterobacteriaceae
    Salmonella
    Gonococcal
    Legionnaires' bacillus
    Other
      Brucellosis
      Typhoid fever
      Tularemia
Mycobacterial
  Tuberculosis
  Leprosy
Spirochetal
  Syphilis (congenital, secondary, or late)
  Leptospirosis
  Relapsing fever (*Borrelia* species)
Mycotic
  Histoplasmosis
  Coccidioidomycosis
  Blastomycosis
  Nocardiosis
  Cryptococcosis
  Candidiasis
  Actinomycosis
Parasitic (e.g., malaria, toxoplasmosis, amebiasis, schisto-
    somiasis, others)
Rickettsial (e.g., Q fever)

Toxins
Industrial toxins (e.g., carbon tetrachloride, yellow phos-
    phorus, trichloroethylene)
Plant toxins
  Mushrooms (e.g., *Amanita phalloides*)
  Aflatoxin

Drug-induced Liver Disease, Including Hepatitis
Drugs implicated in the etiology of chronic hepatitis
  Acetaminophen
  Aspirin

Dantrolene
Ethanol
Isoniazid
Methyldopa
Nitrofurantoin
Oxyphenisatin
Perhexiline maleate
Propylthiouracil
Sulfonamides
Specific classes of drugs associated with acute and/or
    chronic liver dysfunction
  Anesthetics
    Chloroform
    Halothane
    Enflurane
    Methoxyflurane
    Cyclopropane
  Analgesics, anti-inflammatory agents
    Acetaminophen
    Salicylates
    Propoxyphene
    Phenylbutazone
    Indomethacin
    Ibuprofen
    Naproxen
  Antibacterial agents
    Erythromycin
      Estolate
      Ethylsuccinate
      Lactobionate
    Tetracyclines
    Nitrofurantoins
    Sulfonamides
    Penicillin
    Oxacillin
    Cloxacillin
    Carbenicillin
    Chloramphenicol
    Clindamycin
  Antituberculous agents
    Isoniazid
    Rifampin
    Ethionamide
    Para-aminosalicylic acid
    Pyrazinamide
  Antifungal, antiparasitic agents
    Antimony
    Arsenic

    Thiobendazole
    Hycanthone
    5-Fluorocytosine
    Quinacrine
Anticonvulsants
    Phenytoin
    Valproic acid
    Trimethadione
Antihypertensives, diuretics
    Chlorothiazide
    Furosemide
    Chlorthalidone
    Methyldopa
    Hydralazine
Antiarrhythmic agents
    Quinidine
    Aprindine
    Procainamide
Antimetabolites
    6-Mercaptopurine
    Methotrexate
    Azathioprine
    6-Thioguanine
    Chlorambucil
    5-Fluorouracil
    Nitrogen mustard
    Cyclophosphamide
Hormones
    Androgens (e.g., methyltestosterone)
    Corticosteroids
    Estrogens
Oral hypoglycemics
    Chlorpropamide
    Tolbutamide
    Tolazamide
    Acetohexamide
Antithyroid drugs
    Methimazole
    Carbimazole
    Propylthiouracil
Psychoactive agents
    Phenothiazines (especially chlorpromazine)
    Imipramine
    Benzodiazepines
    Meprobamate
    Monoamine oxidase inhibitors
Others
    Doxapram

Cimetidine
Perhexiline maleate
Cinchophen
Gold salts
Allopurinol
Pyridium
Papaverine
Oxyphenisatin
Nicotinic acid
Disulfiram

Others
Autoimmune chronic active hepatitis
Wilson's disease
Granulomatous hepatitis of unknown etiology
Hepatitis associated with systemic disorders
  Hyperthermia
  Cardiac failure
  Shock
  Burns
  Hyperthyroidism
  Hypoxia

References
1. MacGregor IL: Industrial and Environmental Toxins. In general reference 14, p 723.
2. Ockner RK: Drug-induced Liver Disease. In general reference 14, p 691.
3. Koff RS: Viral Hepatitis. In general reference 13, p 326.
4. Patwardhan RV, Tomaiolo PP: Alcohol-and-Drug-Induced Liver Disease. In general reference 13, p 356.

6-P. Cirrhosis, Chronic Liver Disease

Alcoholic
Infectious
  Viral hepatitis (especially B and non-A, non-B)
  Schistosomiasis
  Other infections (uncommon) (e.g., congenital syphilis,
    brucellosis)
Biliary
  Primary biliary cirrhosis
  Primary sclerosing cholangitis
  Secondary biliary cirrhosis (chronic extrahepatic obstruc-
    tion)
Autoimmune chronic active hepatitis
"Cryptogenic" cirrhosis
  Posthepatitic
  Postnecrotic
Chemical
  Toxins
    Alcohol
    Carbon tetrachloride
    Dimethylnitrosamine
    Phosphorus
    Vinyl chloride
    Arsenic
    Beryllium
    Pesticides
  Drugs
    Halothane
    Isoniazid
    Methotrexate
    Methyldopa
    Monamine oxidase inhibitors
    Nitrofurantoin
    Oxyphenisatin
Congestive
  Severe chronic right heart failure
    Tricuspid insufficiency
    Constrictive pericarditis
    Cor pulmonale
    Mitral stenosis
  Hepatic vein obstruction (Budd-Chiari syndrome)
Hereditary or familial disorders
  Hepatolenticular degeneration (Wilson's disease)
  Cystic fibrosis
  Alpha$_1$-antitrypsin deficiency
  Hemochromatosis

    Galactosemia
    Glycogen storage diseases
    Hereditary fructose intolerance
    Tyrosinosis
    Hypervitaminosis A
    Thalassemia (secondary iron overload)
    Sickle cell disease
    Osler-Rendu-Weber syndrome
    Abetalipoproteinemia
Others
    Sarcoidosis
    Granulomatous cirrhosis
    Congenital hepatic fibrosis
    Indian childhood cirrhosis
    Nutritional (e.g., jejunoileal bypass surgery)

References

1. Galambos JT: Cirrhosis. In Smith LH (Ed): *Major Problems in Internal Medicine.* Philadelphia: Saunders, 1979, vol. 17.
2. General reference 14.
3. Tomaiolo PP, Patwardhan RV: Consequences of Chronic Liver Disease. In general reference 13, p 384.

6-Q. Ascites

Without Peritoneal Disease
Portal hypertension
  Cirrhosis (see 6-P)
  Alcoholic hepatitis
  Hepatic congestion
    Congestive heart failure
    Tricuspid insufficiency
    Constrictive pericarditis
    Inferior vena cava obstruction
    Hepatic vein obstruction (Budd-Chiari syndrome)
  Portal vein occlusion
    Thrombosis
    Tumor
  Idiopathic tropical splenomegaly
  Partial nodular transformation
  Hypervitaminosis A
  Fulminant hepatic failure
  Idiopathic
Hypoalbuminemia
  Cirrhosis (see 6-P)
  Nephrotic syndrome
  Protein-losing enteropathy
  Lymphangiectasia
  Severe malnutrition
Miscellaneous
  Myxedema
  Hepatocellular carcinoma (usually with cirrhosis)
  Ovarian disease
    Tumor (Meigs's syndrome)
    Struma ovarii
    Ovarian overstimulation syndrome
  Pancreatic ascites
  Bile ascites
  Chylous ascites
    Rupture (traumatic, surgical) of abdominal lymphatics
    Congenital lymphangiectasia
    Obstructed lymphatics (especially secondary to malig-
        nancy, tuberculosis, filariasis)
    Constrictive pericarditis
    Cirrhosis

With Peritoneal Disease
Infection
  Mycobacterial

Bacterial
  Primary (spontaneous bacterial peritonitis [SBP] in cir-
    rhosis)
  Secondary (ruptured viscus)
Fungal (rare, especially candidiasis, histoplasmosis,
    cryptococcosis)
Parasitic (rare), especially schistosomiasis, ascariasis,
    enterobiasis
Neoplasm
  Primary mesothelioma
  Metastatic carcinomatosis
    Ovarian
    Pancreatic
    Gastric
    Colonic
    Lymphoma
Miscellaneous
  Peritoneal vasculitides
    Systemic lupus erythematosus
    Henoch-Schönlein purpura
    Köhlmeier-Degos disease
  Eosinophilic peritonitis
  Familial Mediterranean fever
  Pseudomyxoma peritonei
  Whipple's disease
  Granulomatous peritonitis
    Foreign bodies (especially starch)
    Sarcoidosis
  Gynecologic lesions (especially endometriosis, ruptured
    dermoid cyst)
  Peritoneal lymphangiectasis

References
1. Bender MD, Ockner RK: Diseases of the Peritoneum,
   Mesentery, and Diaphragm. In general reference 12, p
   1569.
2. Boyer TD: Portal Hypertension and Its Complications. In
   general reference 14, p 464.

6-R. Ascitic Fluid Characteristics in Various Disease States[a]

Condition	Gross appearance	Protein (gm/dl)[b]	RBCs (>10,000/mm³)	Cell count	
				WBCs	Other
Hepatic cirrhosis	Straw-colored or bile-stained	<2.5 (95%)[a]	1%	<250/mm³ (90%)[a]; predominantly endothelial	pH gradient < 0.1[c]
Congestive heart failure	Straw-colored	Variable, 1.5–5.3	10%	<1000/mm³ (90%); usually mesothelial, mononuclear	
Nephrogenic ascites	Straw-colored or chylous[d]	<2.5 (100%)	Unusual	<250/mm³; mesothelial, mononuclear	
Neoplasm	Straw-colored, hemorrhagic, mucinous, or chylous[d]	>2.5 (75%)	20%	>1000/mm³ (50%); variable cell types	Cytology, cell block, peritoneal biopsy
Peritonitis, bacterial	Turbid or purulent	If purulent, >2.5	Unusual	>500/mm³ with >250 neutrophils/mm³	Gram's stain, culture; pH gradient > 0.1[c]

| Peritonitis, tuberculous[d] | Clear, turbid, hemorrhagic, or chylous[d] | >2.5 (50%) | 7% | >1000/mm³ (70%); usually >70% lymphocytes | Peritoneal biopsy, stain and culture for acid-fast bacilli |
| Pancreatic ascites[d] | Turbid, hemorrhagic, or chylous[d] | Variable, often >2.5 | Variable, may be blood-stained | Variable | ↑↑ amylase in ascitic fluid, ↑ in serum |

[a]Since the conditions of examining and selecting patients were not identical in each series, the percentage figures (in parentheses) should be taken as an indication of the order of magnitude rather than as the precise incidence of any abnormal finding. Modified from Glickman RM, Isselbacher KJ: Abdominal Swelling and Ascites. In Isselbacher KJ, et al (Eds): *Harrison's Principles of Internal Medicine* (11th ed). New York: McGraw-Hill, 1987, p 190. Copyright © 1987 by McGraw-Hill Book Co.

[b]Ascitic fluid is generally classified as transudative if the protein content < 2.5 gm/dl and the serum-fluid albumin gradient > 1.1 gm/dl, and as exudative if protein > 2.5 gm/dl and serum-fluid albumin gradient < 1.1 gm/dl. Transudates are usually found in cirrhosis, in congestive heart failure, and with nephrotic ascites; exudates, in neoplastic states and with peritonitis and pancreatic ascites.

[c]pH gradient = blood pH − ascitic fluid pH.

[d]If ascitic fluid is chylous (milky in appearance), then triglyceride content determination and lipoprotein electrophoresis should be performed.

7 GENITOURINARY SYSTEM

7-A. Hematuria

Pseudohematuria (Dyes and Pigments)
Beets
Food dyes
Phenolphthalein
Rifampin
Pyridium
Urates
Porphyrins
Myoglobin
Free hemoglobin (intravascular hemolysis)

Renal Parenchymal Causes
Primary glomerulopathy
   Postinfectious glomerulonephritis
   Benign recurrent hematuria
   Berger's disease (IgA nephropathy)
   Membranoproliferative glomerulonephritis
   Focal glomerulosclerosis
   Crescentic glomerulonephritis
Multisystem and hereditary diseases
   Diabetes mellitus
   Lupus erythematosus

Goodpasture's syndrome
Polyarteritis nodosa, other vasculitides
Endocarditis, shunt nephritis
Hemolytic-uremic syndrome
Henoch-Schönlein purpura
Malignant hypertension
Polycystic kidney disease
Hereditary nephritis (Alport's syndrome)
Fabry's disease
Nail-patella syndrome
Other
Exercise
Pyelonephritis, acute
Nephrolithiasis
Renal cyst
Renal trauma
Renal neoplasm
Coagulopathy, thrombocytopenia
Interstitial nephritis, acute
Analgesic nephropathy
Sickle cell trait or disease
Medullary sponge kidney
Lymphomatous or leukemic infiltration
Hydronephrosis
Oxaluria
Vascular anomalies, intrarenal arteriovenous fistula
Acute febrile illnesses (especially malaria, yellow fever,
    smallpox)
Papillary necrosis
Renal infarction (acute renal artery occlusion, renal vein
    thrombosis)
Renal transplant rejection

Lower Urinary Tract Causes

Congenital anomalies (e.g., ureterocele)
Neoplasms (bladder, ureter, prostate, urethral), benign or
    malignant
Cystitis, prostatitis, urethritis
Calculi
Trauma
Foreign body
Coagulopathy
Varices (renal pelvis, ureter, bladder)
Radiation cystitis
Drugs (especially cyclophosphamide, anticoagulants)
Schistosomiasis
Genitourinary tuberculosis

Non–Urinary Tract Causes
Neoplasm of adjacent organs
Diverticulitis
Pelvic inflammatory disease
Appendicitis

Reference
1. Glassock RJ, Adler SG, Ward HJ, Cohen AH: Primary Glomerular Diseases. In general reference 15, p 929.

7-B. Polyuria

Central diabetes insipidus (see 4-H)
Renal disease
  Nephrogenic diabetes insipidus, congenital
  Chronic renal insufficiency (especially tubulointerstitial disease)
  Diuretic phase of acute renal failure
  Postobstructive diuresis, partial or intermittent obstruction
  Hypercalcemic nephropathy
  Hypokalemic nephropathy
  Sickle cell trait or disease
  Multiple myeloma
  Amyloidosis
  Sarcoidosis
  Sjögren's syndrome
  Decreased protein intake
Osmotic diuresis
  Diabetes mellitus, poorly controlled
  Mannitol or urea administration
  Iodinated contrast dye
  Hyperalimentation
  Tube feedings
Drugs
  Alcohol
  Diuretics
  Lithium
  Demeclocycline
  Methicillin
  Gentamicin
  Amphotericin B
  Phenothiazines
  Sulfonylurea compounds
  Phenytoin

Propoxyphene
Methoxyflurane
Colchicine
Vinblastine
Clonidine
Norepinephrine
Narcotic antagonists
Water load
Psychogenic polydipsia
Intravenous fluid therapy
Drug-induced polydipsia (e.g., phenothiazines, anticho-
linergics)
Resorption of edema fluid

Reference
1. Berl T, Schrier RW: Disorders of Water Metabolism. In
general reference 16, p 1.

7-C. Proteinuria

Benign/Physiologic
Fever
Exercise
Orthostatic
Contrast dye

Usually Non-nephrotic
Chronic pyelonephritis
Other interstitial nephritis (acute or chronic)
Arteriolar nephrosclerosis
Malignant hypertension
Interstitial nephritis
Acute tubular necrosis
Urinary tract obstruction
Nephrolithiasis
Renal neoplasm
Renal trauma
Polycystic kidney disease
Hereditary nephritis (Alport's syndrome)
Glomerular disease, especially:
IgA nephropathy (Berger's disease)
Crescentic glomerulonephritis
Hemolytic-uremic syndrome
Scleroderma
Genitourinary tuberculosis

Often Nephrotic
Primary renal disease, especially:
  Minimal change disease
  Membranous glomerulopathy
  Membranoproliferative glomerulonephritis
  Focal glomerulosclerosis
Systemic disease, especially:
  Diabetes mellitus
  Lupus erythematosus
  Polyarteritis nodosa
  Wegener's granulomatosis
  Henoch-Schönlein purpura
  Mixed cryoglobulinemia
  Amyloidosis (primary or secondary)
  Neoplasm
    Solid tumors (especially lung, colon, stomach, breast)
    Hodgkin's disease, other lymphomas
    Multiple myeloma
  Sarcoidosis
  Myxedema
  Graves' disease
  Sickle cell disease
Toxins, drugs
  Gold
  Mercury
  Heroin
  Nonsteroidal anti-inflammatory drugs
  Tolbutamide, chlorpropamide
  Rifampin
  Probenecid
  Penicillamine
  Captopril
  Trimethadione and other anticonvulsants
  Lithium
Allergens
  Pollens
  Poison ivy and oak
  Snake venom
  Bee or insect stings
  Antitoxin (e.g., tetanus toxoid)
Infection, especially:
  Bacterial (e.g., streptococcal, staphylococcal)
  Hepatitis B
  Cytomegalovirus
  Epstein-Barr virus (infectious mononucleosis)
  Acquired immunodeficiency syndrome (AIDS)
  Syphilis
  Malaria

    Helminthic (e.g., schistosomiasis)
    Leprosy
Miscellaneous
    Congestive heart failure
    Tricuspid insufficiency
    Constrictive pericarditis
    Preeclampsia
    Renal vein thrombosis, inferior vena cava obstruction
    Massive obesity
    Hereditary diseases, especially:
        Congenital nephrotic syndrome
        Alport's syndrome
        Fabry's disease
        Alpha$_1$-antitrypsin deficiency
        Nail-patella syndrome

Reference
1. Glassock RJ, Adler SG, Ward HJ, Cohen AH: Primary Glomerular Diseases. In general reference 15, p 929.

7-D. Glomerulopathy

Primary Renal Disease
Minimal change disease
Membranous glomerulopathy
Membranoproliferative glomerulonephritis
Focal glomerulosclerosis
Crescentic glomerulonephritis
Mesangial proliferative glomerulonephritis (e.g., IgA nephropathy)

Infection
Bacterial, especially:
    Streptococcal
    Endocarditis
    Shunt infection
    Septicemia, especially pneumococcal or staphylococcal
    Meningitis
Viral, especially:
    Hepatitis
    Mononucleosis
    Rubella
    Varicella
    Mumps

Cytomegalovirus
Acquired immunodeficiency syndrome (AIDS)
Syphilis
Parasitic infestation (especially malaria)
Tuberculosis

Systemic Disease
Diabetes mellitus
Lupus erythematosus
Scleroderma
Rheumatoid arthritis
Mixed connective tissue disease
Polyarteritis nodosa
Wegener's granulomatosis
Hemolytic-uremic syndrome
Thrombotic thrombocytopenic purpura
Mixed cryoglobulinemia
Goodpasture's syndrome
Waldenström's macroglobulinemia
Amyloidosis
Neoplasm
Solid tumors (especially lung, stomach, colon, breast)
Hodgkin's disease, other lymphoma
Multiple myeloma, light chain nephropathy
Sarcoidosis
Preeclampsia
Postpartum renal failure
Sickle cell disease
Hepatic cirrhosis

Drugs, Toxins
Mercury
Gold
Penicillamine
Probenecid
Heroin
Amphetamines
Trimethadione
Sulfonamides

Other
Radiation
Hereditary nephritis (Alport's syndrome)
Fabry's disease
Nail-patella syndrome
Congenital nephrotic syndrome
Renal transplant rejection

References
1. Glassock RJ, Adler SG, Ward HG, Cohen AH: Primary Glomerular Diseases. In general reference 15, p 929.
2. Glassock RJ, Cohen AH, Adler SG, Ward HG: Secondary Glomerular Diseases. In general reference 15, p 1014.

7-E. Interstitial Nephropathy

Infection
  Bacterial (pyelonephritis, acute or chronic)
  Mycoplasmal
  Toxoplasmosis
  Leptospirosis
  Brucellosis
  Mononucleosis
  Legionnaires' disease
Urinary tract obstruction, vesicoureteral reflux
Papillary necrosis
Drugs
  Analgesics (especially aspirin, phenacetin)
  Methicillin and penicillin analogues
  Cephalosporins
  Tetracycline
  Rifampin
  Amphotericin B
  Furosemide
  Thiazides
  Nonsteroidal anti-inflammatory agents
  Allopurinol
  Phenytoin
  Azathioprine
  Lithium
  Phenindione
  Warfarin
  Para-aminosalicylic acid
  Polymyxins
Heavy metals
  Lead
  Cadmium
  Uranium
  Copper
  Beryllium
Oxalate deposition
  Hereditary
  Small-bowel disease or resection

Ethylene glycol intoxication
Methoxyflurane anesthesia
Uric acid deposition
  Gout
  Chemotherapy of leukemia or lymphoma
Hypercalcemia, e.g.:
  Hyperparathyroidism
  Neoplasm, multiple myeloma
  Milk-alkali syndrome
  Sarcoidosis
Hypokalemia
Radiation
Neoplastic disease
  Multiple myeloma
  Light chain nephropathy
  Leukemic or lymphomatous infiltration
  Waldenström's macroglobulinemia
Vascular causes
  Arteriolar nephrosclerosis
  Renal artery stenosis
  Atheroembolic disease
  Sickle cell trait or disease
Hereditary causes
  Hereditary nephritis
  Medullary sponge kidney
  Medullary cystic disease
  Polycystic kidney disease
  Cystinosis
  Fabry's disease
Systemic lupus erythematosus
Mixed cryoglobulinemia
Sarcoidosis
Sjögren's syndrome
Amyloidosis
Balkan nephropathy
Transplant rejection

Reference

1. Cotran RS, Rubin RH, Tolkoff-Rubin NE: Tubulointerstitial Diseases. In general reference 15, p 1143.

7-F. Renal Tubular Acidosis

Distal
Pyelonephritis, chronic
Obstructive uropathy
Drugs, toxins
   Amphotericin B
   Analgesics
   Toluene
   Lithium
   Cyclamate
Nephrocalcinosis, especially:
   Primary hyperparathyroidism
   Vitamin D intoxication
   Primary hypercalciuria
   Medullary sponge kidney
   Hyperthyroidism
Autoimmune diseases
   Hypergammaglobulinemic states, especially:
      Hyperglobulinemic purpura
      Cryoglobulinemia
      Familial hypergammaglobulinemia
   Systemic lupus erythematosus
   Sjögren's syndrome
   Thyroiditis
   Chronic active hepatitis
   Primary biliary cirrhosis
   Diffuse interstitial pulmonary fibrosis
Genetically transmitted diseases
   Sickle cell disease
   Ehlers-Danlos syndrome
   Hereditary elliptocytosis
   Fabry's disease
   Wilson's disease
   Medullary cystic disease
   Hereditary fructose intolerance
Hepatic cirrhosis
Balkan nephropathy
Oxalate nephropathy
Multiple myeloma
Renal transplantation
Idiopathic (sporadic or hereditary)

Proximal
Primary (sporadic or hereditary)
Transient (infants)

Carbonic anhydrase deficiency (e.g., genetic or acetazol-
    amide-induced)
Fanconi syndrome (multiple proximal tubular defects)
    Drugs and toxins
        Outdated tetracycline
        Toluene
        Gentamicin
        Streptozotocin
        Lead
        Cadmium
        Mercury
    Multiple myeloma
    Amyloidosis
    Sjögren's syndrome
    Vitamin D–deficient, dependent, and resistant states
    Cystinosis
    Tyrosinemia
    Lowe's syndrome
    Wilson's disease
    Hereditary fructose intolerance
    Pyruvate carboxylase deficiency
    Medullary cystic disease
    Paroxysmal nocturnal hemoglobinuria
    Osteopetrosis
    Renal transplantation

Other
Mineralocorticoid deficiency
    Adrenal insufficiency (see 4-G)
    Congenital enzyme defects (e.g., 21-hydroxylase defi-
        ciency)
    Isolated aldosterone deficiency (e.g., familial, heparin-in-
        duced)
    Hyporeninemic hypoaldosteronism
        Diabetes mellitus
        Tubulointerstitial disease (e.g., nephrosclerosis)
        Nonsteroidal anti-inflammatory drugs
Mineralocorticoid-resistant states ("pseudohypoaldosteron-
    ism")
    Drugs
        Spironolactone
        Triamterene
        Amiloride
    Obstructive uropathy
    Sickle cell disease
    Acute interstitial nephritis (e.g., methicillin-induced)

Renal transplantation
Distal tubular dysfunction secondary to chronic glomerular
    disease

References
1. Cogan MG, Rector FC: Acid-Base Disorders. In general
   reference 15, p 457.
2. Kaehny WD, Gabow PA: Pathogenesis and Management
   of Metabolic Acidosis and Alkalosis. In general reference
   16, p 141.

7-G. Urinary Tract Obstruction

Urethral
Congenital urethral stenosis, web, atresia
Posterior urethral valves
Inflammation or stricture
Trauma

Bladder Neck
Prostatic hypertrophy, prostatitis
Carcinoma (prostate, bladder)
Bladder infection
Functional
    Neuropathy (peripheral neuropathy, spinal cord injury or
        trauma)
    Drugs (parasympatholytics, ganglionic blockers)

Ureteral
Ureteral-pelvic junction stricture
Intraureteral
    Clots
    Stones
    Crystals (e.g., sulfa, uric acid)
    Papillae (necrosed)
    Trauma (edema, stricture)
    Tumor
    Foreign bodies
Extraureteral
    Endometriosis
    Retroperitoneal tumor or metastases, especially:
        Cervical
        Endometrial
        Ovarian
        Prostatic

> Lymphoma
> Sarcoma
Fibrosis
> Idiopathic
> Associated with inflammation, drugs (e.g., methyser-
> gide), radiation, inflammatory bowel disease
Pregnancy
Aortic or iliac aneurysm
Surgical ligation
Retroperitoneal hemorrhage

References
1. Brenner BM, Humes HD: Urinary Tract Obstruction. In general reference 1, p 1353.
2. Wilson DR, Schrier RW: Obstructive Nephropathy: Pathophysiology and Management. In general reference 16, p 495.

7-H. Nephrolithiasis

Calcium-Containing Stones
Idiopathic
Primary hypercalciuria (absorptive, renal-leak) with or without hyperuricosuria
Hypercalcemic states (see also 1-L)
> Primary hyperparathyroidism
> Malignancy
> Immobilization
> Milk-alkali syndrome
> Vitamin D excess
> Sarcoidosis
> Hyperthyroidism
Renal tubular acidosis, distal
Medullary sponge kidney
Carbonic anhydrase inhibitors (e.g., acetazolamide)
Cushing's disease or syndrome
Hypoparathyroidism
Hyperoxaluria
> Primary (congenital)
> Increased metabolic production (e.g., ethylene glycol or methoxyflurane excess)
> Increased gastrointestinal absorption
>> Increased dietary intake

Small-bowel disease or resection (e.g., jejunoileal bypass, celiac sprue, regional enteritis)

Magnesium Ammonium Phosphate Stones (Struvite)
Chronic infection (usually with urea-splitting organisms,
e.g., *Proteus, Klebsiella, Pseudomonas*), especially
associated with:
  Chronic Foley catheter use
  Ileal loop

Uric Acid and/or Xanthine Stones
Gout
Leukemia, lymphoma (especially after chemotherapy)
Purine pathway enzyme deficiency states
  Lesch-Nyhan syndrome
  Glycogen storage disease
  Xanthinuria
Drugs (e.g., aspirin, probenecid)
Gastrointestinal disorders associated with chronic diarrhea
  (especially with ileostomy)

Cystine Stones
Cystinuria

Reference
1. Smith LH: Urolithiasis. In Schrier RW, Gottschalk CW
(Eds): *Diseases of the Kidney* (4th ed). Boston: Little,
Brown, 1988, p 785.

7-I. Acute Renal Failure

Prerenal Azotemia
Hypovolemia
  Hemorrhage
  Gastrointestinal losses
  Sweating
  Diuretic use
  Third-spacing (e.g., intestinal ileus)
  Burns
Decreased effective circulating volume
  Cirrhosis/ascites, hepatorenal syndrome
  Nephrotic syndrome
  Cardiac causes (e.g., congestive heart failure, acute
    myocardial infarction, pericardial tamponade)
Catabolic states, e.g.:
  Starvation with stress
  Sepsis, serious infection
  Postsurgical state
  Steroids
  Tetracycline
Breakdown of blood in gastrointestinal tract or resorption of
    hematoma

Drugs, Toxins
Heavy metals
  Mercury
  Arsenic
  Lead
  Cadmium
  Uranium
  Bismuth
  Copper
  Platinum
Carbon tetrachloride, other organic solvents
Ethylene glycol
Pesticides
Fungicides
X-ray contrast media
Antibiotics
  Penicillin
  Tetracycline
  Aminoglycosides
  Cephalosporins
  Amphotericin B
  Sulfonamides
  Rifampin

Polymyxin
Other drugs
    Nonsteroidal anti-inflammatory agents
    Captopril
    Phenytoin
    Phenindione
    Methoxyflurane
    Furosemide
    EDTA

Ischemic Disorders
Major trauma, surgery
Massive hemorrhage, severe volume depletion
Pancreatitis
Septic shock
Crush injury
Hemolysis, transfusion reaction
Rhabdomyolysis

Glomerular/Vascular Diseases
Poststreptococcal glomerulonephritis
Systemic lupus erythematosus
Scleroderma
Polyarteritis nodosa, hypersensitivity angiitis
Henoch-Schönlein purpura
Bacterial endocarditis
Serum sickness
Goodpasture's syndrome
Crescentic glomerulonephritis, idiopathic
Wegener's granulomatosis
Drug-induced vasculitis
Malignant hypertension
Hemolytic-uremic syndrome
Thrombotic thrombocytopenic purpura
Preeclampsia
Abruptio placentae
Postpartum renal failure
Transplant rejection

Interstitial/Intratubular Diseases
Interstitial nephritis (see 7-E), especially:
    Infection
    Drugs
    Oxalate deposition
    Hypercalcemia
Pyelonephritis, papillary necrosis
Hyperuricemia

Hypercalcemia
Radiation

Major Vessel Diseases
Renal artery thrombi, emboli, stenosis
Renal vein or inferior vena cava thrombosis
Dissecting aneurysm (aorta with or without renal arteries)

Postrenal Causes*
Urethral obstruction
Bladder neck obstruction
Ureteral obstruction

References
1. Levinsky NG, Alexander EA, Venkatachalam MA: Acute Renal Failure. In general reference 15, p 1181.
2. Schrier RW, Conger JD: Acute Renal Failure: Pathogenesis, Diagnosis, and Management. In general reference 16, p 423.

*See 7-G.

7-J. Renal Failure, Reversible Factors

Infection
Obstruction
Volume depletion
Drugs, toxins
Congestive heart failure
Hypertension
Pericardial tamponade
Hypercalcemia
Hyperuricemia (> 15–20 mg/dl)
Hypokalemia

Reference
1. Alfrey AC: Chronic Renal Failure: Manifestations and Pathogenesis. In general reference 16, p 461.

7-K. Urinary Diagnostic Indices[a]

	Prerenal azotemia	Oliguric acute renal failure
Urine osmolality (mOsm/kg H_2O)	>500	<350
Urine Na^+ (mEq/L)	<20	>40
Urine/plasma urea nitrogen	>8	<3
Urine/plasma creatinine	>40	<20
Fractional excretion of Na^+ (%)[b]	<1	>1

[a]These indices are useful only in oliguric states.

[b]Fractional excretion of Na^+ =

$$\frac{\text{(urine } Na^+ \text{ concentration) (plasma creatinine concentration)}}{\text{(plasma } Na^+ \text{ concentration) (urine creatinine concentration)}} \times 100\%.$$

Source: Modified from Miller TR, Anderson RJ, Linas SL, et al: Urinary Diagnostic Indices in Acute Renal Failure: A Prospective Study. *Ann Intern Med* 89:49, 1978.

7-L. Chronic Renal Failure

Glomerulopathy, Primary Renal*

Glomerulopathy Associated with Systemic Disease*

Genetically Transmitted Disease
Polycystic kidney disease
Hereditary nephritis
Fabry's disease
Oxalosis
Cystinosis
Medullary cystic disease
Medullary sponge kidney
Nail-patella syndrome
Congenital nephrotic syndrome

Vascular Diseases
Nephrosclerosis
Malignant hypertension
Cortical necrosis
Renal artery stenosis, thrombosis, emboli
Renal vein thrombosis, inferior vena cava thrombosis

Interstitial Disease†
Drugs: analgesics, lithium, amphotericin B
Heavy metals: lead, cadmium, beryllium

Urinary Tract Obstruction‡

References
1. General reference 15.
2. General reference 16.

*See 7-D.
†See 7-E.
‡See 7-G.

7-M. Indications for Dialysis

Chemical Criteria
Volume overload
Serum K^+ > 6 mEq/L (despite medical management)
Serum HCO_3^- < 10 mEq/L, pH < 7.20
Blood urea nitrogen > 100–200 mg/dl
Serum creatinine > 10–20 mg/dl

Symptomatic Criteria
Central nervous system symptoms (e.g., lethargy, confusion, seizures, asterixis)
Gastrointestinal symptoms (e.g., nausea, vomiting)
Pericarditis
Bleeding diathesis

Miscellaneous Indications (Conditions Not Necessarily Associated with Renal Failure)
Hypercalcemia
Hypermagnesemia
Hyperuricemia
Hypernatremia
Hypothermia
Removal of drugs or toxins

Reference
1. Shinaberger JH: Indications for Dialysis. In Massry SG, Sellers AL (Eds): *Clinical Aspects of Uremia and Dialysis.* Springfield, Ill.: Thomas, 1976, p 490.

7-N. Impotence

Aging
Psychogenic causes
Testicular causes (primary or secondary)
    Congenital hypogonadism (especially Froehlich's syndrome, Klinefelter's syndrome, hypogonadotropic eunuchoidism)
    Acquired hypogonadism
      Viral orchitis
      Trauma
      Radiation
      Hepatic insufficiency
      Chronic pulmonary disease
      Chronic renal failure
      Granulomatous disease (especially leprosy)
    Testicular carcinoma
    Pituitary tumor, especially when associated with hyperprolactinemia
    Pituitary insufficiency
Neurologic disease
    Anterior temporal lobe lesion
    Spinal cord disease (e.g., multiple sclerosis)
    Loss of sensory input
      Diabetes mellitus
      Polyneuropathy
      Tabes dorsalis
      Dorsal root ganglia disease
    Lesions of nervi erigentes
      Aortic bypass surgery
      Total prostatectomy
      Rectosigmoid surgery
Drugs
    Estrogens
    Anticholinergic agents
    Antidepressants (e.g., amitriptyline, doxepin)
    Antihypertensive agents
      Guanethidine
      Methyldopa
      Clonidine
      Reserpine
      Propranolol
      Thiazides
      Spironolactone
    Antipsychotic agents (e.g., phenothiazines, haloperidol, thioridazine)

Tranquilizers (e.g., diazepam, chlordiazepoxide, barbiturates)
  Addictive drugs (e.g., heroin, methadone)
Alcoholism
Vascular disease (e.g., Leriche syndrome)
Priapism, previous
Penile disease
  Trauma
  Peyronie's disease

Reference
1. Walsh PC, Wilson JD: Impotence and Infertility in Men. In general reference 1, p 217.

7-O. Menorrhagia and Nonmenstrual Vaginal Bleeding

Ovulatory Bleeding
Midcycle ovulatory bleeding (normal variant)
Inadequate corpus luteum (luteal phase defect)
Uterine or endometrial disease
  Endometritis
  Endometriosis
  Uterine adenomyosis
  Endometrial polyps
  Uterine leiomyomas
  Carcinoma
  Intrauterine synechiae
  Intrauterine device
Vaginal or cervical disease
  Vaginitis, cervicitis
  Cervical scarring
  Carcinoma

Anovulatory
Estrogen withdrawal bleeding
Estrogen breakthrough bleeding
  Chronic, continuous estrogen therapy
  Polycystic ovarian disease
  Estrogen-secreting ovarian tumor

Progesterone breakthrough bleeding (e.g., continuous low-
dose oral contraceptives)
Abortion
Ectopic pregnancy
Ovarian destructive lesions (e.g., tumor, chronic salpingo-
oophoritis)
Hypothalamic or pituitary lesion (e.g., tumor, sarcoidosis)
Adrenal disease (hyper- or hypofunction)
Thyroid disease (hyper- or hypofunction)
Stress, psychogenic factors

References
1. Carr BR, Wilson JD: Diseases of the Ovary and Female
   Reproductive Tract. In general reference 1, p 1818.
2. Riddick DH: Disorders of Menstrual Function. In Danforth
   DN, Scott JR (Eds): *Obstetrics and Gynecology* (5th
   ed). Philadelphia: Lippincott, 1986, p 873.

8 HEMATOLOGIC SYSTEM

8-A. Anemia—Hypoproliferative (Low Reticulocyte Count)

Nutrient Deficiency
Iron deficiency
  Chronic blood loss
  Pregnancy
  Dietary deficiency
  Malabsorption
    Subtotal gastrectomy
    Malabsorption syndromes
  Hemoglobinuria/hemosiderinuria
    Intravascular hemolysis
  Hemodialysis
Vitamin B_{12} deficiency
  Dietary deficiency (rare)
  Impaired absorption
    Insufficient intrinsic factor
      Pernicious anemia
      Gastrectomy (total or partial)
      Gastric mucosal injury (e.g., lye ingestion)
      Congenital
    Malabsorption syndromes
      Sprue, tropical or nontropical

        Ileal resection
        Regional ileitis
        Infiltrative intestinal disease (e.g., lymphoma)
        Chronic pancreatitis
        Familial selective malabsorption
        Drug-induced malabsorption
      Competitive absorption
        Diphyllobothrium latum (fish tapeworm)
        Blind-loop syndromes
    Increased requirements
      Pregnancy
      Neoplasia
Folate deficiency
    Dietary deficiency (especially alcoholics, infants)
    Impaired absorption
      Malabsorption syndromes
        Sprue, tropical or nontropical
        Whipple's disease
        Small-intestinal resection
        Infiltrative intestinal disease (e.g., lymphoma)
        Scleroderma
        Amyloidosis
      Drug-induced malabsorption (anticonvulsants)
    Increased requirements
      Pregnancy
      Infancy
      Hemolytic anemia
      Chronic exfoliative dermatitis
      Neoplasia
      Uremia
    Impaired metabolism
      Trimethoprim
      Methotrexate
      Pyrimethamine
      Alcohol
Other nutritional deficiencies
    Vitamin A
    Pyridoxine (rare)
    Vitamin C
    Starvation
    Protein deficiency (kwashiorkor)

Anemia of Chronic Disease
Chronic infection
    Subacute bacterial endocarditis
    Osteomyelitis
    Chronic pyelonephritis
    Chronic pulmonary infection

Tuberculosis
Chronic fungal infection
Pelvic inflammatory disease
Chronic inflammatory diseases
Rheumatoid arthritis
Rheumatic fever
Systemic lupus erythematosus
Vasculitis
Inflammatory bowel disease
Acquired immunodeficiency syndrome (AIDS)/AIDS related complex
Malignancy
Chronic renal disease
Chronic liver disease
Endocrine dysfunction
Hypothyroidism
Adrenal insufficiency
Panhypopituitarism
Hyperparathyroidism

Bone Marrow Disorders
Congenital
Red cell aplasia (Diamond-Blackfan anemia)
Congenital dyserythropoietic anemias
Hereditary sideroblastic anemias
Aplastic
Pancytopenia (see 8-L)
Pure red cell aplasia
Congenital (Diamond-Blackfan anemia)
Acquired
Associated with thymoma, chronic lymphocytic leukemia, etc.
Drug-induced
Toxic
Megaloblastic
Antimetabolites (e.g., 5-fluorouracil, 6-thioguanine, 6-mercaptopurine, azathioprine)
Sideroblastic (e.g., alcohol, lead, isoniazid, chloramphenicol)
Aplastic (see 8-L)
Infiltrative, with or without fibrosis
Infection
Tuberculosis
Fungal disease
Gaucher's and other lipid storage diseases
Malignancy
Hematologic (leukemia, lymphoma, myeloma)
Marrow metastases

Neoplastic
  Leukemia, acute and chronic
  Lymphoproliferative disorders
    Lymphoma, with marrow involvement
      Hodgkin's disease
      Non-Hodgkin's lymphoma
    Plasma cell myeloma
    Hairy-cell leukemia
  Myeloproliferative disorders
    Agnogenic myeloid metaplasia with fibrosis
    Essential thrombocythemia
    Chronic myelogenous leukemia
  Myelodysplastic syndromes
    Refractory anemia (RA)
    RA with ringed sideroblasts
    RA with excess of blasts (RAEB)
    RAEB in transformation
    Chronic myelomonocytic leukemia

Other
Marathon runner's anemia (physiologic)

References

1. Erslev AJ: Anemia of Chronic Renal Failure; Anemia of Endocrine Disorders; Anemia of Chronic Disorders. In general reference 18, pp 417, 425, 522.
2. Beck WS: The Megaloblastic Anemias. In general reference 18, p 434.
3. Fairbanks VF, Beutler E: Iron Deficiency. In general reference 18, p 466.
4. Wintrobe MM et al: The Anemia of Chronic Disorders. In general reference 17, p 646.
5. Herbert V: Hematologic Complications of Alcoholism I, II. *Semin Hematol*, vol. 17, 1980.
6. Dressendorfer RH, Wade CE, Amsterdam EA: Development of Pseudoanemia in Marathon Runners During a 20-day Road Race. *JAMA* 246:1215, 1981.
7. Jandl JH (Ed): *Blood. Textbook of Hematology.* Boston: Little, Brown, 1987.

8-B. Anemia—Hyperproliferative (Increased Reticulocyte Count)

Blood Loss

Hypersplenism

Hemolytic Anemia
Hereditary
  Membrane abnormalities
    Hereditary spherocytosis
    Hereditary elliptocytosis
    Hereditary stomatocytosis
    Acanthocytosis (abetalipoproteinemia)
    Others
  Enzyme deficiencies
    Glucose 6-phosphate dehydrogenase
    Pyruvate kinase
    Others
  Hemoglobinopathies
    Qualitative
      Sickle-cell anemia
      Hemoglobin C disease
      Unstable hemoglobin disease
      Others
    Unbalanced chain synthesis
      Thalassemias
Acquired
  Nonimmune
    Traumatic
      Prosthetic valves and other cardiac abnormalities
      March hemoglobinuria
      Burns
    Microangiopathic hemolytic anemia
      Disseminated intravascular coagulation
      Thrombotic thrombocytopenic purpura
      Hemolytic uremic syndrome
      Vasculitis
      Malignant hypertension
    Infectious agents
      Malaria
      Clostridium perfringens
      Bartonella
      Babesiosis
      Others
    Chemical agents
      Naphthalene

Arsine
Copper
Chlorates
Venoms
Distilled water (IV)
Others
Paroxysmal nocturnal hemoglobinuria
Hypophosphatemia
"Spur cell" anemia (liver disease)
Immune
Warm antibody mediated
Incompatible blood transfusion
Hemolytic disease of newborn
Idiopathic
Secondary
Infectious
Viral (e.g., Epstein-Barr virus, cytomegalovirus)
Collagen-vascular disorders
Systemic lupus erythematosus
Rheumatoid arthritis
Malignancy
Lymphoproliferative disorders
Solid tumors
Other
Sarcoidosis
Inflammatory bowel disease
Drugs (many)
Cold antibody mediated
Idiopathic
Secondary
Infectious
Viral (e.g., Epstein-Barr virus)
Mycoplasma pneumoniae
Malignancy
Paroxysmal cold hemoglobinuria

References
1. Wintrobe MM, et al: Introduction to the Hemolytic Anemias. In general reference 17, p 734.
2. Beutler E: Glucose-6-phosphate Dehydrogenase Deficiency. In general reference 18, p 561.
3. Packman CH, Leddy JP: Acquired Hemolytic Anemia due to Warm-reacting Autoantibodies; Cryopathic Hemolytic Syndromes; Drug-related Immunologic Injury of Erythrocytes. In general reference 18, pp 632, 642, 647.

8-C. Polycythemia

Spurious
    Decreased plasma volume (e.g., dehydration, burns)
    "Stress" erythrocytosis (Gaisböck's syndrome)
Secondary
    Appropriate (associated with tissue hypoxia)
        Decreased arterial PO_2
            Altitude
            Chronic pulmonary disease
            Alveolar hypoventilation
            Cyanotic congenital heart disease
        Normal arterial PO_2
            Carboxyhemoglobinemia (e.g., cigarette smoking)
            Hemoglobinopathies (with an increased affinity for
                oxygen)
            Cobalt ingestion
    Inappropriate
        Renal disorders
            Hydronephrosis
            Renal cysts
            Renal cell carcinoma
        Endocrine disorders
            Cushing's syndrome
            Primary hyperaldosteronism
            Pheochromocytoma
            Androgen therapy
        Hepatoma
        Cerebellar hemangioblastoma
        Uterine leiomyoma
        Familial erythrocytosis
Primary
    Polycythemia rubra vera

References
1. Wintrobe MM et al: Polycythemia: Erythrocytosis. In general reference 17, p 991.
2. Erslev AJ: Erythrocyte Disorders—Erythrocytosis. In
   general reference 18, p 673.

D. Granulocytopenia

Infections
  Viral
    Influenza
    Infectious mononucleosis
    Infectious hepatitis
    Rubella
    Chickenpox
    Smallpox
    Poliomyelitis
    Others
  Bacterial
    Overwhelming bacteremia
    Typhoid fever
    Tularemia
    Brucellosis
  Mycobacterial
    Miliary tuberculosis
  Rickettsial
  Protozoan
    Malaria
Chemical agents, drugs, physical agents
  Predictable
    Antineoplastic agents
    Benzene
    Ionizing radiation
  Idiosyncratic
    Aminopyrine
    Phenothiazines
    Antithyroid drugs
    Sulfonamides
    Anticonvulsants
    Antibiotics
    Ethanol
    Others
Systemic illness
  Systemic lupus erythematosus
  Felty's syndrome
  Acquired immunodeficiency syndrome (AIDS)/AIDS re-
    lated complex
Hypersplenism
Nutritional
  B_{12} or folate deficiency
  Cachexia
  Alcoholism

Bone marrow dysfunction
  Acute leukemias (aleukemic)
  Lymphoproliferative disorders
  Myelofibrosis
    Primary—myeloproliferative disorders
    Secondary
      Tumor infiltration
      Infection
  Aplastic anemia
  Myelodysplastic syndromes
Immune neutropenia
  Drug-induced
  Collagen vascular disease (systemic lupus erythemato-
    sus)
  Neoplasia
  Autoimmune neutropenia
Other
  Benign neutropenia of blacks
  Chronic idiopathic neutropenia
  Cyclic neutropenia
  Benign familial neutropenia

References
1. Finch SC: Neutropenia. In general reference 18, p 773.
2. Budman DR, Steinberg AD: Hematologic Aspects of Systemic Lupus Erythematosus. *Ann Intern Med* 86:220,
   1977.
3. Spivak JL, Bender BS, Quinn TC: Hematologic Abnormalities in the Acquired Immune Deficiency Syndrome.
   Am J Med 77:224, 1984.

8-E. Granulocytosis

Reactive
Infection
   Bacterial (primarily)
   Mycobacterial
   Fungal
   Rickettsial
   Viral
   Spirochetal
   Parasitic
Physical stimuli
   Exercise
   Trauma
   Seizures
Inflammation, acute and chronic
   Collagen vascular disorders
   Hypersensitivity reactions
   Gout
   Vasculitis
   Nephritis
   Inflammatory bowel disease
   Hepatitis
   Pancreatitis
   Dermatitis
Neoplasm
Tissue necrosis
   Myocardial infarction
   Gangrene
   Burns
Drugs, toxins, especially:
   Corticosteroids
   Epinephrine
   Lithium
   Endotoxin
   Histamine
   Lead
Hematologic disorders
   Hemorrhage
   Postsplenectomy, functional asplenia
   Recovery from agranulocytosis
   Hemolytic anemia
   Bone marrow infiltration (e.g., solid tumor, tuberculosis)
Metabolic disorders
   Diabetic ketoacidosis
   Cushing's syndrome
   Eclampsia

Uremia
   Thyroid storm
Pregnancy

Autonomous
Myeloproliferative disorders
   Chronic myelogenous leukemia
   Polycythemia rubra vera
   Agnogenic myeloid metaplasia
   Essential thrombocythemia
Acute leukemia

Congenital Causes

Reference
1. Finch SC: Neutrophilia. In general reference 18, p 794.

8-F. Lymphocytosis

Infections
   Viral
      Infectious mononucleosis
      Infectious lymphocytosis
      Cytomegalovirus infection
      Mumps
      Measles
      Chickenpox
      Viral hepatitis
      Others
   Bacterial
      Pertussis
      Brucellosis
      Tuberculosis
   Spirochetal
      Syphilis, secondary and congenital
   Protozoan
      Toxoplasmosis
Hematologic disorders
   Lymphocytic leukemia, acute and chronic
   Non-Hodgkin's lymphoma with marrow involvement
Drug hypersensitivity
   Phenytoin
   p-Aminosalicylic acid
Miscellaneous
   Thyrotoxicosis

Post–cardiopulmonary bypass syndrome
Serum sickness
Immune thrombocytopenic purpura
Immune hemolytic anemia

Reference
1. Cassileth PA: Lymphocytosis. In general reference 18,
   p 950.

8-G. Lymphocytopenia

Immunodeficiency syndromes
   Acquired immunodeficiency syndrome (AIDS)/AIDS re-
      lated complex
   Congenital immunodeficiency syndromes
      Wiskott-Aldrich syndrome
      Ataxia-telangiectasia
      Di George's syndrome
   Common variable immunodeficiency
Increased lymphocyte destruction
   Radiation therapy
   Antineoplastic chemotherapy
   Antilymphocyte/antithymocyte globulin
   Corticosteroid or adrenocorticotropic hormone administra-
      tion or excess
Increased lymphocyte loss
   Thoracic duct drainage
   Intestinal lymphectasia
   Intestinal lymphatic obstruction (e.g., lymphoma)
   Whipple's disease
   Severe right-sided heart failure
      Tricuspid insufficiency
      Constrictive pericarditis
Other
   Sarcoidosis
   Advanced malignancy
   Miliary tuberculosis
   Renal failure
   Aplastic anemia
   Collagen-vascular disorders
      Systemic lupus erythematosus

References
1. Cassileth PA: Lymphocytopenia. In general reference 18,
   p 955.

2. Spivak JL, Bender BS, Quinn TC: Hematologic Abnormalities in the Acquired Immune Deficiency Syndrome. *Am J Med* 77:224, 1984.

8-H. Monocytosis

Infections
  Tuberculosis
  Subacute bacterial endocarditis
  Syphilis
Hematologic disorders
  Myelodysplastic syndromes
  Acute nonlymphocytic leukemia (especially acute monocytic leukemia)
  Myeloproliferative disorders
  Lymphoproliferative disorders
    Hodgkin's disease
    Non-Hodgkin's lymphoma
    Myeloma
  Malignant histiocytosis
  Postsplenectomy
  Recovery from neutropenia
    Infectious
    Drug-induced
    Postchemotherapy
  Benign familial neutropenia
Collagen-vascular disorders
  Rheumatoid arthritis
  Systemic lupus erythematosus
  Temporal arteritis
  Polyarteritis nodosa
  Polymyositis
Malignancy
  Any solid tumor
Gastrointestinal disorders
  Sprue
  Ulcerative colitis
  Regional enteritis
Miscellaneous
  Sarcoidosis

Reference

1. Cassileth PA: Monocytosis. In general reference 18, p 861.

8-I. Eosinophilia

Infections
    Bacterial
        Scarlet fever
        Tuberculosis
        Leprosy
        Others
    Parasitic
        Protozoans (e.g., toxoplasmosis, amebiasis, malaria)
        Metazoans (e.g., trichinosis, filariasis, schistosomiasis)
        Arthropods (e.g., scabies)
Allergic disorders
    Hay fever
    Asthma
    Bronchopulmonary aspergillosis
    Urticaria
    Angioneurotic edema
    Serum sickness
    Food allergy
Skin disorders
    Psoriasis
    Eczema
    Erythema multiforme
    Dermatitis herpetiformis
    Exfoliative dermatitis
    Pityriasis rosea
    Ichthyosis
    Pemphigus vulgaris
    Facial granuloma
Drug reactions
Hematologic disorders
    Myeloproliferative disorders
    Lymphoproliferative disorders
    Acute nonlymphocytic leukemia
    Myelodysplastic syndromes
    Postsplenectomy
    Hypereosinophilic syndrome
Malignancy
    Advanced solid tumors
Collagen-vascular disorders
    Rheumatoid arthritis
    Polyarteritis nodosa
    Vasculitis
    Dermatomyositis
    Systemic lupus erythematosus
    Eosinophilic fasciitis

Gastrointestinal disorders
  Eosinophilic gastroenteritis
  Ulcerative colitis
  Regional enteritis
Others
  Adrenal insufficiency
  Loeffler's syndrome
  Chronic eosinophilic pneumonia
  Sarcoidosis
  Radiation therapy
  Chronic renal disease
  Familial eosinophilia

References
1. Zucker-Franklin D: Eosinopenia and Eosinophilia. In general reference 18, p 825.
2. Chusid MJ, Dale DC, West BC, Wolff SM: The Hypereosinophilic Syndrome. *Medicine* 54:1, 1975.
3. Pearson DJ, Rosenow EC: Chronic Eosinophilic Pneumonia (Carrington's): A Follow-up Study. *Mayo Clin Proc* 53:73, 1978.

8-J. Thrombocytopenia

Decreased Production
Primary hematologic disorders
  Aplastic anemia
  Acute leukemia
  Lymphoproliferative disorders
    Lymphoma
    Myeloma
    Chronic lymphocytic leukemia
  Myeloproliferative disorders
    Agnogenic myeloid metaplasia with myelofibrosis
    Chronic myelogenous leukemia (accelerated phase)
  Myelodysplastic syndromes
  Selective megakaryocytic aplasia
Bone marrow infiltration
  Solid tumor
  Infection
    Tuberculosis
    Other
  Gaucher's disease
  Osteopetrosis

Drugs
  Selective megakaryocytic suppression
    Thiazides
    Alcohol
    Estrogens
    Interferon
  Nonselective myelosuppression
    Predictable (e.g., antineoplastic chemotherapy)
    Idiosyncratic (e.g., phenylbutazone)
Cyclic thrombocytopenia
Nutritional deficiency
  Folate
  Vitamin B_{12}
  Iron (rare)
Viral infections
  Influenza
  Rubella
  Infectious mononucleosis
  Thai hemorrhagic fever
  Dengue fever
  Others
Paroxysmal nocturnal hemoglobinuria
Hereditary disorders
  Wiskott-Aldrich syndrome
  May-Hegglin anomaly
Congenital causes
  Fanconi's anemia
  Amegakaryocytic thrombocytopenia with congenital mal-
    formations
  Congenital rubella or cytomegalovirus infection
  Maternal thiazide ingestion

Increased Destruction
Congenital—nonimmune
  Erythroblastosis fetalis
  Maternal preeclampsia
  Congenital viral infection
  Giant cavernous hemangioma
Congenital—immune
  Maternal drug ingestion
  Isoimmune neonatal thrombocytopenia
  Maternal autoimmune thrombocytopenic purpura
Acquired—nonimmune
  Infections
    Bacterial
      Sepsis
      Typhoid fever

Viral
  Infectious mononucleosis
  Cytomegalovirus
  Herpes
Malaria
Rickettsial
  Rocky Mountain spotted fever
Toxic shock syndrome
Microangiopathic hemolytic anemia
  Disseminated intravascular coagulation
  Thrombotic thrombocytopenic purpura
  Hemolytic-uremic syndrome
  Vasculitis
Drugs
Extracorporeal circulation
Anaphylaxis
Acquired—immune
  Drug-induced
    Quinine/quinidine
    Gold salts
    Heparin
    Thiazides
    Sulfonamides
    Indomethacin
    Others
  Neoplasia-associated
    Lymphoproliferative disorders
    Solid tumors
  Collagen-vascular disorders
    Systemic lupus erythematosus
    Rheumatoid arthritis
  Acquired immunodeficiency syndrome (AIDS)/AIDS re-
    lated complex
  Posttransfusion purpura
  Idiopathic autoimmune thrombocytopenic purpura
    Acute
    Chronic
  Sarcoidosis
  Hashimoto's thyroiditis
  Hyperthyroidism

Sequestration/Dilution
Hypersplenism
Hypothermia
Extracorporeal circulation
Massive blood transfusion

References
1. Aster RH: Thrombocytopenia Due to Diminished or Defective Platelet Production; Thrombocytopenia Due to Enhanced Platelet Destruction; Thrombocytopenia Due to Sequestration of Platelets; Thrombocytopenia Due to Platelet Loss. In general reference 18, pp 1290, 1298, 1338, 1340.
2. Burns TR, Saleem A: Idiopathic Thrombocytopenic Purpura. *Am J Med* 75:1001, 1983.

8-K. Thrombocytosis

Primary
Myeloproliferative disorders
  Essential thrombocythemia
  Polycythemia vera
  Chronic myelogenous leukemia
  Agnogenic myeloid metaplasia with myelofibrosis

Secondary
Chronic inflammatory disorders
  Collagen-vascular disorders
    Rheumatoid arthritis
    Polyarteritis nodosa
    Wegener's granulomatosis
    Other vasculitis
  Chronic infections
    Tuberculosis
    Osteomyelitis
    Others
  Acute infections
  Inflammatory bowel disease
    Ulcerative colitis
    Regional ileitis
  Sarcoidosis
  Hepatic cirrhosis
Malignancy
Acute hemorrhage
Iron deficiency
Hemolytic anemia
Splenectomy
Recovery from thrombocytopenia (rebound)
  Myelosuppressive drug–induced
  Vitamin B_{12} or folate deficiency
  Alcohol-induced

Reference
1. Williams WJ: Thrombocytosis. In general reference 18, p 1342.

8-L. Pancytopenia

Aplastic anemias
  Congenital
    Fanconi's anemia
  Drug/chemical-induced
    Benzene
    Chloramphenicol
    Phenylbutazone
    Gold salts
    Cytotoxic chemotherapy
    Alcohol
    Others
  Radiation exposure
  Idiopathic
  Infection
    Viral, especially hepatitis
  Immunologic
Hematologic neoplasia
  Leukemia (aleukemic)
  Lymphoproliferative disorders
    Lymphoma with marrow involvement
    Plasma cell myeloma
    Hairy-cell leukemia
  Myeloproliferative disorders
    Agnogenic myeloid metaplasia with myelofibrosis
  Myelodysplastic syndromes
Marrow infiltration/replacement
  Infection
    Tuberculosis
    Fungal
  Gaucher's and other lipid storage diseases
  Solid tumor
  Osteopetrosis
Nutritional deficiencies
  Vitamin B_{12}
  Folate
Other
  Collagen vascular diseases
    Systemic lupus erythematosus

Acquired immunodeficiency syndrome (AIDS)/AIDS re-
lated complex
Paroxysmal nocturnal hemoglobinuria
Hypersplenism
Bacterial sepsis
Viral infection
Sarcoidosis

References
1. Wintrobe MM, et al: Pancytopenia, Aplastic Anemia, and
   Pure Red Cell Aplasia. In general reference 17, p 698.
2. Erslev AJ: Aplastic Anemia. In general reference 18,
   p 151.

8-M. Lymphadenopathy

Benign
Infection
  Bacterial (any)
    Mycobacterial
  Fungal
  Viral
  Protozoal
  Rickettsial
  Chlamydial
Local inflammation
  Trauma
  Dermatitis
Hypersensitivity reaction
  Serum sickness
  Drug reaction
    Phenytoin
Collagen-vascular disorders
  Systemic lupus erythematosus
  Rheumatoid arthritis
  Dermatomyositis
Endocrine disorders
  Hyperthyroidism
Acquired immunodeficiency syndrome (AIDS)/AIDS related
    complex
Sarcoidosis
Other
  Mucocutaneous lymph node syndrome
  Angioimmunoblastic lymphadenopathy
  Autoimmune hemolytic anemia

Malignant
Acute leukemia
Lymphoproliferative disorders
   Lymphoma
   Plasma cell myeloma
   Chronic lymphocytic leukemia
   Hairy-cell leukemia
Myeloproliferative disorders
   Chronic myelogenous leukemia
   Agnogenic myeloid metaplasia
Solid tumors

Reference
1. Weinstein IM: Lymph Node Enlargement and Splenomegaly. In general reference 18, p 937.

8-N. Splenomegaly

Infection
   Bacterial
   Viral
   Rickettsial
   Fungal
   Protozoal
Inflammatory
   Collagen-vascular disorders
   Hypersensitivity reactions
      Serum sickness
      Drug reactions
Hematologic neoplasms
   Acute leukemia
   Lymphoproliferative disorders
      Lymphoma
      Chronic lymphocytic leukemia
      Hairy-cell leukemia
   Myeloproliferative diseases
   Myelodysplastic syndromes
Nonmalignant hematologic disorders
   Autoimmune hemolytic anemia
   Congenital hemolytic anemias
      Hemoglobinopathies
      Hereditary spherocytosis
   Megaloblastic anemias
   Iron-deficiency anemia
   Angioimmunoblastic lymphadenopathy

Congestive splenomegaly
  Portal hypertension
  Splenic or portal vein compression or thrombosis
  Congestive heart failure
  Budd-Chiari syndrome
Infiltrative disorders
  Gaucher's and other lipid storage diseases
  Histiocytic disorders
  Amyloidosis
  Metastatic solid tumors
Other
  Acquired immunodeficiency syndrome (AIDS)/AIDS re-
      lated complex
  Sarcoidosis
  Splenic trauma/hemorrhage
  Splenic cysts
  Splenic abscess

References
1. Wintrobe MM, et al: Disorders Primarily Involving the
   Spleen. In general reference 17, p 1426.
2. Jandl JH: The Spleen and Hypersplenism. In Jandl JH,
   Blood. Boston: Little, Brown, 1987, p 407.

8-O. Disorders of Hemostasis

Platelet Disorders
Quantitative platelet disorders (see 8-J)
Qualitative platelet disorders
  Congenital
    Bernard-Soulier syndrome
    Glanzmann's thrombasthenia
    Storage pool deficiencies
    Von Willebrand's disease
  Acquired
    Uremia
    Myeloproliferative disorders
    Myelodysplastic syndromes
    Dysproteinemias
    Drug-induced
      Aspirin
      Nonsteroidal anti-inflammatory agents
      Dextran
      Hydroxyethyl starch
      Dipyridamole
      Sulfinpyrazone
      Others
    Extracorporeal circulation

Coagulation Disorders
Congenital
  Factor deficiencies
    VIII (hemophilia A)
    IX (hemophilia B)
    XI
    V
    VII
    X
    II
    Combined deficiency of vitamin K–dependent factors
  Fibrinogen disorders
    Afibrinogenemia
    Hypofibrinogenemia
    Dysfibrinogenemia
  Von Willebrand's disease
Acquired
  Vitamin K deficiency
    Malabsorption syndromes
    Broad-spectrum antibiotic therapy
    Cholestatic jaundice
    Dietary deficiency

Hemorrhagic disease of the newborn
Oral anticoagulant use/abuse
Factor X deficiency and amyloidosis
Circulating anticoagulants
Factor VIII
Associated with hemophilia A
Autoimmune disorders
Lymphoproliferative disorders/dysproteinemias
Pregnancy
Drug therapy
Penicillin
Factors IX and others
Lupus anticoagulant
With Factor II deficiency
Consumptive coagulopathies
Disseminated intravascular coagulation
Liver disease
Acquired dysfibrinogenemia
Fibrinolytic states
Heparin administration
Massive blood transfusion

References

1. Weiss HJ: Congenital Qualitative Platelet Disorders; Acquired Qualitative Platelet Disorders. In general reference 18, pp 1346, 1355.
2. Furie B: Disorders of the Vitamin K–dependent Coagulation Factors; Acquired Anticoagulants. In general reference 18, pp 1421, 1424.
3. Ratnoff OD, Forbes CD: *Disorders of Hemostasis.* Orlando: Grune & Stratton, 1984.

8-P. Hypercoagulable States

Congenital
Antithrombin III deficiency
Protein C deficiency
Protein S deficiency
Homocystinuria
Dysfibrinogenemias

Acquired
Oral contraceptive use
Lupus anticoagulant
Myeloproliferative disorders
    Essential thrombocythemia
    Polycythemia vera
Paroxysmal nocturnal hemoglobinuria
Heparin-associated thrombocytopenia
Prothrombin complex concentrate infusion
Nephrotic syndrome
Pregnancy
Disseminated intravascular coagulation (DIC)
Thrombotic thrombocytopenic purpura
Malignancy (with DIC)
Sickle cell anemia
Hyperviscosity syndromes
Previous venous thrombosis
Venous trauma

References
1. Jandl JH: Thrombotic and Fibrinolytic Disorders. In Jandl JH (Ed): *Blood*. Boston: Little, Brown, 1987, p 1141.
2. Schafer AI: The Hypercoagulable States. *Ann Intern Med* 102:814, 1985.

8-Q. Disorders of Immunoglobulin Synthesis

Hypogammaglobulinemia
Congenital
  X-linked agammaglobulinemia
  Selective IgA deficiency
  Severe combined immunodeficiency
Acquired
  Common variable immunodeficiency
  Lymphoproliferative disorders
    Plasma cell myeloma
    Lymphoma
    Chronic lymphocytic leukemia
  Radiation therapy
  Antineoplastic chemotherapy
  Associated with thymoma

Hypergammaglobulinemia
Polyclonal
  Chronic inflammatory disease
    Chronic infections
    Collagen-vascular disorders
    Malignancy
    Hepatic cirrhosis
    Chronic active hepatitis
    Acquired immunodeficiency syndrome (AIDS)/AIDS related complex
    Inflammatory bowel disease
    Sarcoidosis
    Others
  Angioimmunoblastic lymphadenopathy
Monoclonal
  Lymphoproliferative malignancies
    Plasma cell myeloma
    Non-Hodgkin's lymphoma
    Chronic lymphocytic leukemia
    Macroglobulinemia
    Heavy chain diseases
  Amyloidosis
  Monoclonal gammopathy of undetermined significance

References
1. Rosen FS: Immunodeficiency Diseases. In general reference 18, p 957.
2. Bergsagel DE: Plasma Cell Neoplasms—General Considerations. In general reference 18, p 1067.

9 INFECTIOUS DISEASE

9-A. Fever of Unknown Origin in the United States*

Infection†
Bacterial
  Sinusitis
  Bacterial endocarditis
  Intravascular catheter infections
  Osteomyelitis
  Upper abdominal cause
    Cholangitis
    Cholecystitis
    Empyema of gallbladder
    Pancreatic, hepatic, splenic, subphrenic abscess
  Lower abdominal cause
    Appendiceal abscess
    Diverticulitis
    Pelvic inflammatory disease or abscess
    Perirectal abscess
    Peritonitis
  Urinary tract cause
    Perinephric, intrarenal, or prostatic abscess
    Pyelonephritis (rare)
    Ureteral obstruction

Bacteremia without primary focus, especially:
  Meningococcemia
  Gonococcemia
  Salmonellosis
  Listeriosis
  Brucellosis
  Yersiniosis
  Tularemia
  Leptospirosis
  Syphilis
Tuberculosis
Viral (e.g., Epstein-Barr virus [infectious mononucleosis],
  hepatitis, Coxsackie B, cytomegalovirus, acquired im-
  munodeficiency syndrome [AIDS]/AIDS-related com-
  plex)
Chlamydial, rickettsial (e.g., psittacosis, Q fever)
Parasitic, protozoan, especially:
  Amebiasis
  Trichinosis
  Malaria
  Toxoplasmosis
Fungal, especially:
  Histoplasmosis
  Blastomycosis
  Cryptococcosis
  Coccidioidomycosis

Malignancy†
Leukemia, lymphoma
Solid tumor, especially carcinoma of:
  Kidney
  Lung
  Pancreas
  Liver
  Colon
  Metastatic carcinoma
Atrial myxoma

Collagen-Vascular Disease†
Lupus erythematosus
Rheumatoid arthritis
Rheumatic fever
Polyarteritis nodosa, hypersensitivity vasculitis
Wegener's granulomatosis
Temporal arteritis

Drugs
Antibiotics, especially:

    Penicillins
    Cephalosporins
    Sulfonamides
    Amphotericin B
Allopurinol
Phenytoin
Barbiturates
Iodides
Methyldopa
Procainamide
Quinidine
Propylthiouracil

Other
Pulmonary emboli, multiple
Thrombophlebitis
Sarcoidosis
Hepatitis, granulomatous or alcoholic
Inflammatory bowel disease
Whipple's disease
Thyroiditis
Thyrotoxicosis
Trauma with hematoma in enclosed space (e.g., peri-
    splenic, perivesical)
Myelofibrosis
Hemolytic states
Dissecting aneurysm
Fabry's disease
Familial Mediterranean fever
Gout
Addison's disease
Weber-Christian disease
Cyclic neutropenia
Thermoregulatory disorders
Factitious fever
Habitual hyperthermia

References
1. Petersdorf RG, Root RK: Chills and Fever. In general reference 1, p 50.
2. Jacoby GA, Swartz MN: Current Concepts: Fever of Undetermined Origin. *N Engl J Med* 289:1407, 1973.

*Defined as temperature of > 38.3°C daily for 2 to 3 weeks, with
cause undiagnosed despite 1 week of intensive studies in hospital.
†Infection, malignancy, and collagen-vascular disease ultimately account for about 75% of fevers of unknown origin.

9-B. Most Common Organisms Causing Specific Infections

Infection	Organisms
Skin infection	
Burns	*Staphylococcus aureus*, Enterobacteriaceae, *Pseudomonas* sp., *Serratia* sp., *Providencia* sp.
Decubiti	*S. aureus*, group A streptococci, anaerobic streptococci, Enterobacteriaceae, *Pseudomonas* sp.
Wounds (traumatic and surgical)	*S. aureus*, group A streptococci, Enterobacteriaceae, *Clostridium perfringens*, *Clostridium tetani*
Bites—Human	Viridans streptococci, group A streptococci, *S. aureus*, *Bacteroides* sp., *Fusobacterium* sp.
Bites—Cat	*Pasteurella multocida*, *S. aureus*
Bites—Dog	Viridans streptococci, *S. aureus*, *S. epidermidis*, *P. multocida*, *Bacteroides* sp., *Fusobacterium* sp.
Meningitis	Viruses, pneumococci, meningococci, group A streptococci, *Haemophilus influenzae*, Enterobacteriaceae, *Pseudomonas* sp., *Listeria monocytogenes*, *S. aureus*

Condition	Organisms
Otitis media	Pneumococci, *H. influenzae, Branhamella catarrhalis, S. aureus,* group A streptococci
Conjunctivitis	Adenovirus, enterovirus, *H. influenzae,* pneumococci, group A streptococci, *Neisseria, Chlamydia trachomatis*
Keratitis	*Pseudomonas* sp., pneumococci, *S. aureus, Neisseria gonorrhoeae, Neisseria meningitidis,* herpes simplex, fungi (*Fusarium, Aspergillus, Candida*), *Acanthamoeba* (associated with contact lens)
Sinusitis	Pneumococci, *H. influenzae,* group A streptococci, anaerobes, viruses, *Bacteroides* sp., peptostreptococci, *Fusobacterium* sp.
Pharyngitis	Viruses, group A streptococci, *Corynebacterium hemolyticus*
Laryngitis	Respiratory viruses, group A streptococci, *B. catarrhalis*
Bronchitis	Respiratory syncytial virus, adenovirus, *Mycoplasma pneumoniae,* pneumococci, *H. influenzae, B. catarrhalis,* staphylococci
Pneumonia	Respiratory viruses, pneumococci, group A streptococci, *H. influenzae, Klebsiella* and other gram-negative bacilli, *S. aureus, M. pneumoniae, Legionella pneumophila*
Lung abscess	*Bacteroides* sp., peptostreptococci, *Fusobacterium* sp., *S. aureus, Klebsiella pneumoniae,* anaerobes, *Pseudomonas aeruginosa, Streptococcus pyogenes*
Endocarditis Acute	*S. aureus, Staphylococcus epidermidis,* pneumococci, groups A and D streptococci, Enterobacteriaceae, diphtheroids, *Candida albicans,* and other fungi

9-B. Most Common Organisms Causing Specific Infections (continued)

Infection	Organisms
Subacute	Viridans streptococci, *Streptococcus bovis*, enterococci, *Haemophilus parainfluenzae*, *Haemophilus aphrophilus*, fungi, especially *Candida* and *Aspergillus*
Septic thrombophlebitis	*S. aureus*, *S. epidermidis*, *Candida sp.*, *Pseudomonas sp.*, Enterobacteriaceae
Gastroenteritis	Enteric viruses, *Escherichia coli*, *Salmonella*, *Shigella*, *Campylobacter*, *S. aureus*
Peritonitis	Enterobacteriaceae, enterococci, *Bacteroides*, group A streptococci, pneumococci, *S. aureus*, *Clostridium sp.*
Urinary tract infections Cystitis, pyelonephritis	Herpes simplex, *Chlamydia trachomatis*, Enterobacteriaceae, *Staphylococcus saprophyticus*, gonococci, *Pseudomonas*, enterococci, *Mycobacterium tuberculosis*
Urethritis	*Chlamydia trachomatis*, gonococci, Herpes simplex
Vaginitis	Viruses, *Chlamydia*, *Candida sp.*, *Trichomonas*, *Gardnerella vaginalis*, *Bacteroides sp.*, peptococci, *Treponema pallidum*
Pelvic inflammatory disease—salpingitis	*N. gonorrhoeae*, *Chlamydia*, Enterobacteriaceae, *Bacteroides*, *Mycoplasma*, streptococci

Epididymitis—orchitis	Enterobacteriaceae, *N. gonorrhoeae, C. trachomatis, M. tuberculosis*
Prostatitis	Enterobacteriaceae (*E. coli*), *Pseudomonas,* gonococci, *S. aureus,* enterococci
Septicemia	*E. coli* and other gram-negative bacilli, *S. aureus, S. epidermidis,* pneumococci, groups A and D streptococci, *Bacteroides*
Osteomyelitis	*S. aureus,* group A, B streptococci, Enterobacteriaceae, *Pseudomonas sp., Salmonella sp.*
Arthritis, septic	*S. aureus,* pneumococcus, group A, B streptococci, *H. influenzae,* gonococci, *S. epidermidis,* Enterobacteriaceae

References

1. General reference 19.
2. Sanford JP: *Guide to Antimicrobial Therapy 1987.* W Bethesda, MD: Antimicrobial Therapy Inc, 1987.

9-C. Antimicrobial Drugs of Choice

Organism	Drugs
GRAM-POSITIVE COCCI	
Staphylococcus aureus or epidermidis	Penicillin or penicillinase-resistant penicillin, cephalosporin, vancomycin, clindamycin, imipenem (add aminoglycoside for initial infective endocarditis therapy)
Streptococcus pneumoniae	Penicillin, cephalosporin, erythromycin, chloramphenicol, vancomycin
Streptococcus pyogenes (group A)	Penicillin, erythromycin, a cephalosporin, vancomycin
Enterococcus (group D streptococcus)	Ampicillin or vancomycin (with gentamicin or streptomycin for endocarditis)
Anaerobic streptococcus species	Penicillin G, clindamycin, cephalosporin, chloramphenicol, erythromycin, vancomycin
GRAM-NEGATIVE COCCI	
Neisseria gonorrhoeae	Amoxicillin (with probenecid) or ceftriaxone, penicillin G, cefoxitin, spectinomycin, trimethoprim/sulfamethoxazole (TMP/SMX), chloramphenicol
Neisseria meningitidis	Penicillin G, chloramphenicol, cefuroxime, cefotaxime, sulfonamide (prophylaxis with rifampin)

GRAM-POSITIVE BACILLI

Bacillus anthracis (anthrax)
Penicillin G, erythromycin, tetracycline

Clostridium difficile
Metronidazole or vancomycin, bacitracin

Clostridium perfringens
Penicillin G, chloramphenicol, metronidazole, clindamycin

Clostridium tetani
Penicillin G or a tetracycline, erythromycin

Listeria monocytogenes
Ampicillin with or without gentamicin, TMP/SMX, tetracycline, erythromycin, chloramphenicol, penicillin G

GRAM-NEGATIVE BACILLI

Haemophilus influenzae
Ampicillin, chloramphenicol, cefuroxime, cefotaxime, ceftriaxone (serious infections) TMP/SMX, tetracycline

Escherichia coli
Ampicillin with or without aminoglycoside, cephalothin, cefoxitin, carbenicillin, TMP/SMX, imipenem

Klebsiella pneumoniae
Cefotaxime, aminoglycoside (gentamicin, tobramycin, amikacin), TMP/SMX, imipenem, aztreonam

Enterobacter
Cefotaxime, aminoglycoside, (gentamicin, tobramycin, amikacin), carbenicillin, ticarcillin, piperacillin

Proteus mirabilis
Ampicillin, cephalosporin, aminoglycoside, carbenicillin, ticarcillin

Providencia stuartii
Cefotaxime, imipenem, amikacin, ticarcillin, TMP/SMX

Serratia
Cefotaxime, ceftizoxime, ceftriaxone, gentamicin or amikacin, imipenem, aztreonam, carbenicillin

9-C. Antimicrobial Drugs of Choice (continued)

Organism	Drugs
Pseudomonas aeruginosa	Carbenicillin or ticarcillin, tobramycin, piperacillin, ceftazidime, imipenem or cefoperazone with amikacin, tobramycin, or gentamicin, aztreonam
Salmonella typhosa	Chloramphenicol, amoxicillin, TMP/SMX, ceftriaxone, cefoperazone
Shigella	TMP/SMX, chloramphenicol, ampicillin, tetracycline
Bacteroides fragilis	Clindamycin or metronidazole, cefoxitin, chloramphenicol, ticarcillin or piperacillin, imipenem
Brucella	Tetracycline with or without streptomycin, TMP/SMX, chloramphenicol with or without streptomycin
Bordetella pertussis	Erythromycin, TMP/SMX, ampicillin
Acinetobacter	Imipenem, tobramycin, gentamicin, carbenicillin, TMP/SMX, ceftazidime
Legionella pneumophila	Erythromycin with or without rifampin, tetracycline, TMP/SMX
MISCELLANEOUS	
Mycobacterium tuberculosis	Isoniazid with rifampin, ethambutol, streptomycin, pyrazinamide, aminosalicylic acid (PAS)
Nontuberculous mycobacteria	Isoniazid with rifampin with or without ethambutol, streptomycin, ethionamide, cycloserine, rifabutine (Ansamycin)
Actinomyces israelii	Penicillin G, tetracycline
Nocardia	Trisulfapyrimidines, TMP/SMX, minocycline, ampicillin or erythromycin

Treponema pallidum	Penicillin G, tetracycline, erythromycin
Leptospira	Penicillin G, tetracycline
Mycoplasma pneumoniae	Erythromycin, tetracycline
Rickettsia	Tetracycline, chloramphenicol
Chlamydia trachomatis	Tetracycline, erythromycin, sulfonamide
Pneumocystis carinii	TMP/SMX, pentamidine
Toxoplasma gondii	Pyrimethamine and sulfonamide
Giardia lamblia	Quinacrine, metronidazole, furazolidone
Trichomonas vaginalis	Metronidazole

FUNGI

Aspergillus	Amphotericin B, flucytosine
Blastomyces dermatitidis	Ketoconazole, amphotericin B
Candida albicans	Amphotericin B with or without flucytosine and rifampin (topical: amphotericin B, clotrimazole, econazole, miconazole, nystatin)
Coccidioides immitis	Ketoconazole, amphotericin B (meningitis)
Cryptococcus neoformans	Ketoconazole, amphotericin B, and flucytosine
Histoplasma capsulatum	Ketoconazole, amphotericin B
Sporothrix schenckii	Potassium iodide (topical), amphotericin B

9-C. Antimicrobial Drugs of Choice (continued)

Organism	Drugs
VIRUSES	
Herpes simplex	Acyclovir, vidarabine (topical: trifluridine, vidarabine, idoxuridine).
Human immunodeficiency virus	Zidovudine (azidothymidine or AZT)
Influenza A	Amantadine
Respiratory syncytial virus	Ribavirin
Varicella zoster	Acyclovir, vidarabine

References
1. General reference 19.
2. The Choice of Antimicrobial Drugs. *Med Let*, vol 28 (710):33, 1986.
3. Sanford JP: *Guide to Antimicrobial Therapy 1987*. W Bethesda, MD: Antimicrobial Therapy Inc, 1987.

9-D. Classification of Human Immunodeficiency Virus Infections

Group I. Acute infection (antibody seroconversion)
Group II. Asymptomatic infection
Group III. Persistent generalized lymphadenopathy
Group IV. Other disease

Subgroup A. Constitutional disease
Subgroup B. Neurologic disease
Subgroup C. Secondary infectious diseases
   Category C-1. Specified secondary infectious diseases listed in the Center for Disease Control surveillance definition for AIDS (i.e., *Pneumocystis carinii* pneumonia, cryptosporidiosis, toxoplasmosis, intestinal strongyloidiasis, isosporiasis, candidiasis [esophageal, bronchopulmonary], cryptococcosis, histoplasmosis, *Mycobacterium avium-intracellulare* or *Mycobacterium kansasii,* cytomegalovirus, herpes virus infection)
   Category C-2. Other specified secondary infectious disease (oral hairy leukoplakia, herpes zoster, recurrent *Salmonella* bacteremia, nocardiosis, tuberculosis, candidiasis [thrush])
Subgroup D. Secondary cancers (Kaposi's sarcoma, lymphoreticular malignancies)
Subgroup E. Other conditions

References

1. Classification System for Human T-Lymphotropic Virus Type III/Lymphadenopathy-Associated Virus Infections. *MMWR* 35(20):334, 1986.
2. Fauci AS, et al.: Acquired Immunodeficiency Syndrome: Epidemiologic, Clinical, Immunologic and Therapeutic Considerations. *Ann Intern Med* 100:92, 1984.

9-E. VDRL, Biologic False-Positive

Infection
Spirochetal
  Yaws
  Pinta
  Bejel
  Leptospirosis
  Relapsing fever
  Rat-bite fever
Bacterial
  Pneumococcal pneumonia
  Scarlet fever
  Subacute bacterial endocarditis
  Tuberculosis
  Leprosy
  Chancroid
Viral
  Measles
  Varicella
  Vaccinia
  Hepatitis
  Infectious mononucleosis
  Postimmunization
Mycoplasmal
Chlamydial (lymphogranuloma venereum)
Rickettsial (typhus)
Protozoal (malaria, sleeping sickness)
Filarial
Fungal (coccidioidomycosis)

Noninfectious Causes
Aging
Pregnancy
Drug addiction
Collagen-vascular disease (especially lupus erythematosus, rheumatoid arthritis)
Serum sickness
Thyroiditis
Other hypergammaglobulinemic states
Blood transfusion
Malignancy

Reference
1. Rudolph A: Syphilis. In general reference 19, p 611.

10 INTEGUMENT

10-A. Alopecia

Nonscarring
Physiologic
   Postnatal period
   Pregnancy
   Aging (pattern baldness)
Traction
Drugs
   Cytotoxic agents
   Oral contraceptives
   Heparin
   Coumarin
   Colchicine
   Propranolol
   Levodopa
   Bromocriptine
   Thallium
   Bismuth
   Borax
   Vitamin A (excess)
   Thiouracil
Serious systemic illness, childbirth, other stress

Cutaneous disease
  Seborrheic dermatitis
  Eczema
  Psoriasis
  Cosmetics, other local irritants
Lupus erythematosus
Hypothyroidism
Hypopituitarism
Syphilis, secondary
Nutritional deficiency states (kwashiorkor, marasmus, iron
    deficiency)
Alopecia areata
Hereditary
Congenital

Scarring
Physical and chemical agents
  Burns
  Freezing
  Mechanical trauma
  Acid, alkali
  Radiation
Infection
  Bacterial (including pyogenic infection, tertiary syphilis,
      leprosy, lupus vulgaris)
  Fungal (e.g., ringworm)
  Viral (especially varicella-zoster, variola)
  Protozoal (leishmaniasis)
Systemic disease
  Lupus erythematosus, systemic or discoid
  Scleroderma or morphea
  Sarcoidosis
  Dermatomyositis
  Amyloidosis
  Neoplasm
    Metastatic carcinoma
    Lymphoma
Cutaneous disease
  Basal cell carcinoma
  Lichen planus
  Cicatricial pemphigoid
  Necrobiosis lipoidica diabeticorum
Congenital

Reference
1. Bertolino AP, Freedberg IM: Hair. In general reference
   20, p 627.

10-B. Erythema Multiforme

Infections
    Viral (especially herpes simplex, infectious mononucleo-
        sis)
    Bacterial
    Mycoplasmal
    Chlamydial (lymphogranuloma venereum)
    Fungal (especially histoplasmosis, coccidioidomycosis)
    Parasitic (*Trichomonas,* malaria)
Vaccines (e.g., smallpox, polio, BCG)
Drugs, toxins
    Antibiotics (especially penicillin, sulfonamides, tetracy-
        clines)
    Metals: arsenic, mercury, gold
    Antihistamines
    Barbiturates
    Codeine
    Phenytoin
    Sulfonylureas
    Codeine
    Hydralazine
    Salicylates
    Thiazides
    Phenylbutazone
Neoplasms and hematologic disorders
    Lymphoma
    Leukemia
    Carcinoma
    Multiple myeloma
    Polycythemia vera
Physical factors and contact reactions
    Radiation
    Sunlight
    Cold
    Poison oak
    Fire sponge (*Tedania ignis*)
    Collagen-vascular disease
        Lupus erythematosus, systemic or discoid
        Rheumatoid arthritis
        Polyarteritis nodosa
        Wegener's granulomatosis
        Dermatomyositis
        Reiter's syndrome
Sarcoidosis
Menstruation, pregnancy
Loeffler's syndrome

Beer ingestion
Idiopathic

Reference
1. Elias PM, Fritsch PO: Erythema Multiforme. In general
   reference 20, p 555.

10-C. Erythema Nodosum

Infection
  Bacterial
    Streptococci
    Yersinia
    Cat-scratch fever
    Tularemia
  Fungal
    Histoplasmosis
    Coccidioidomycosis
    Blastomycosis
    Trichophyton
  Tuberculosis
  Leprosy
  Leptospirosis
  Chlamydial (lymphogranuloma venereum, psittacosis)
  Viral
Drugs
  Penicillins
  Sulfonamides
  Salicylates
  Halides
  Oral contraceptives
Sarcoidosis
Behçet's syndrome
Leukemia, lymphoma
Radiation therapy
Inflammatory bowel disease
Idiopathic

Reference
1. Bordi EE, Lazarus GS: Panniculitis. In general reference
   20, p 1131.

10-D. Hirsutism and Generalized Hypertrichosis

Anorexia, malnutrition
Drugs
 Minoxidil
 Corticosteroids
 Androgenic steroids
 Progestins
 Danazol
 Phenytoin
 Diazoxide
 Penicillamine
Endocrine disorders
 Adrenogenital syndrome
 Adrenal hyperplasia, adenoma, carcinoma
 Pituitary tumor (especially Cushing's disease, acromegaly, prolactin-secreting tumor)
 Polycystic ovary syndrome
 Ovarian tumor
 Hypothyroidism
Central nervous system disease
 Encephalitis
 Multiple sclerosis
 Head trauma
Dermatomyositis
Hereditary or congenital conditions
 Cutaneous porphyria
 Hurler's syndrome
 Morquio's disease
 Leprechaunism
 Cornelia de Lange's syndrome
 Hypertrichosis lanuginosa

Reference
1. Bertolino AP, Freedberg IM: Hair. In general reference 20, p 627.

10-E. Maculopapular Eruption, Generalized

Drugs (especially antibiotics)
Infections
  Viral
    Rubeola
    Rubella
    Roseola
    Erythema infectiosum (human parvovirus)
    Infectious mononucleosis
    Cytomegalovirus
    Hepatitis B
    Other viruses (including adeno-, entero-, reo-, arbo-,
      rhabdovirus)
    Live-virus vaccine (e.g., measles)
  Bacterial, especially:
    Streptococcal
    Staphylococcal
    Salmonella
    Meningococcemia, chronic
  Other
    Mycoplasmal
    Syphilis, secondary
    Leptospirosis
    Rat-bite fever
    Rickettsial (e.g., Rocky Mountain spotted fever, murine
      typhus)
    Psittacosis
    Toxoplasmosis
    Trichinosis
Systemic lupus erythematosus
Dermatomyositis
Sarcoidosis
Pityriasis rosea

Reference
1. General reference 20.

10-F. Petechiae and Purpura

Platelet Disorders
Thrombocytopenia (see 8-J)
  Drugs, especially:
    Cytotoxic agents
    Aspirin
    Phenytoin
    Nonsteroidal anti-inflammatory agents
    Quinidine
    Quinine
    Gold
  Disseminated intravascular coagulation
    Overwhelming infection
      Bacterial (especially meningococcal, gonococcal,
        staphylococcal, gram-negative)
      Viral (especially entero-, arbo-, adenovirus, acquired
        immunodeficiency syndrome [AIDS])
      Rickettsial (Rocky Mountain spotted fever, louse-
        borne typhus)
      Miliary tuberculosis
      Malaria
    Anaphylaxis
    Neoplasm (especially leukemia, lymphoma, and carci-
      noma of lung, prostate, or pancreas)
  Thrombotic thrombocytopenic purpura
  Immune thrombocytopenic purpura
  Posttransfusion purpura
  Wiskott-Aldrich syndrome
Functional platelet disorders (e.g., Glanzmann's thrombas-
    thenia, von Willebrand's disease)
Thrombocytosis

Vascular/Extravascular Causes
Vasculitis (palpable purpura)
  Henoch-Schönlein purpura
  Polyarteritis nodosa
  Wegener's granulomatosis
  Lupus erythematosus
  Rheumatoid arthritis
  Subacute bacterial endocarditis
  Hepatitis B
  Serum sickness
  Cryoglobulinemia
  Sjögren's syndrome
  Hyperglobulinemic purpura
  Waldenström's macroglobulinemia

  Lymphoproliferative disorders (especially Hodgkin's disease, lymphosarcoma)
  Drugs
    Antibiotics (penicillin, sulfonamides, tetracycline)
    Thiazides
    Nonsteroidal anti-inflammatory agents
    Hydralazine
    Cimetidine
    Phenytoin
    Allopurinol
    Quinidine
    Propylthiouracil
    Ketoconazole
    Gold
Aging
Prolonged elevated venous pressure or other trauma
Steroids (endogenous or exogenous)
Amyloidosis
Cholesterol embolization
Ehlers-Danlos syndrome
Pseudoxanthoma elasticum
Hereditary hemorrhagic telangiectasia
Scurvy
Progressive pigmentary purpura

Reference

1. Brodin MB, Zucker-Franklin D: The Skin and the Hematopoietic System. In general reference 20, p 1909.

10-G. Pruritus

Pruritus with Diagnostic Skin Lesions
Infestation (especially scabies, lice, fleas)
Xerosis (dry skin) (e.g., secondary to low humidity or excessive bathing)
Infection, especially bacterial, fungal, varicella
Eczematous dermatitis (e.g., atopic, contact)
Urticaria (see 10-J)
Psoriasis
Dermatitis herpetiformis
Bullous pemphigoid
Lichen planus
Miliaria
Mastocytosis
Mycosis fungoides

Pruritus Without Diagnostic Skin Lesions
Infestation, especially:
  Hookworm
  Onchocerciasis
  Ascariasis
  Trichinosis
Drugs
  Opiates
  Aspirin
  Estrogens, progestins, androgens
  Erythromycin
  Sulfonylureas
  Phenothiazines
  Quinidine
  Vitamin B complex
  PUVA
Obstructive liver disease
  Bile duct obstruction, extrahepatic
  Bile duct obstruction, intrahepatic
    Biliary cirrhosis
    Drug-induced cholestasis (oral contraceptives, phenothiazines, chlorpropamide)
    Intrahepatic cholestasis of pregnancy
Neoplasm, especially:
  Lymphoma, leukemia
  Abdominal malignancy
  Central nervous system malignancy
  Carcinoid tumor
Polycythemia vera
Iron deficiency

Diabetes mellitus
Hyperthyroidism
Chronic renal failure (with or without secondary hyperpara-
thyroidism)

Reference
1. Bernhard JD: Clinical Aspects of Pruritus. In general reference 20, p 78.

10-H. Pustules, Generalized

Acne vulgaris
Pyogenic infection (especially disseminated gonococcal)
Viral infection (especially vaccinia, variola)
Syphilis, secondary
Drugs, especially:
  Sulfonamides
  Phenytoin
  Halides
  Corticosteroids
  Androgenic steroids
  Oral contraceptives
Pustular psoriasis
Sweet's syndrome (acute febrile neutrophilic dermatosis)
Behçet's syndrome

Reference
1. General reference 20.

10-I. Telangiectasia

Normal variant (especially with wind or sun exposure)
Endocrine disease
   Chronic liver disease (especially alcoholic cirrhosis)
   Pregnancy, estrogen, or progesterone therapy
   Topical steroid therapy (long-term)
   Hyperthyroidism
Collagen-vascular disease
   Lupus erythematosus, systemic or discoid
   Dermatomyositis
   Rheumatoid arthritis
   Systemic sclerosis, CRST syndrome
Genetically transmitted disease
   Osler-Rendu-Weber syndrome (hereditary hemorrhagic
     telangiectasia)
   Ataxia-telangiectasia
   Fabry's disease
   Xeroderma pigmentosum
States associated with prolonged vasodilatation (e.g., vari-
   cose veins, rosacea, polycythemia vera)
Peripheral vascular disease (e.g., livedo reticularis, ery-
   thema ab igne)
Neoplastic disease, especially:
   Breast cancer
   Bile duct carcinoma
   Carcinoid tumor
   Malignant angioendotheliomatosis
Radiation dermatitis

Reference
1. General reference 20.

10-J. Urticaria

Specific antigen sensitivity (e.g., foods, Hymenoptera
    venom, helminths)
Physical agents
  Pressure, mechanical irritation
  Cold
  Heat
  Light (e.g., sunlight)
Atopic conditions (e.g., allergic rhinitis, asthma)
Drugs
  Opiates, barbiturates
  Antibiotics (especially penicillin, sulfonamides)
  X-ray contrast media
  Nonsteroidal anti-inflammatory agents
  Azo dyes
  Curare
Transfusion of blood or blood components
Vasculitis
  Lupus erythematosus
  Rheumatoid arthritis
  Sjögren's syndrome
  Serum sickness
  Hepatitis B, acute
  Cryoglobulinemia
Mastocytosis (urticaria pigmentosa)
Occult malignancy (especially lymphoma, carcinoma)
Emotional stress
Idiopathic

Reference
1. Soter NA, Wasserman SI: IgE-dependent Urticaria and
  Angioedema. In general reference 20, p 1282.

10-K. Vesicles and Bullae, Generalized

Physical agents
  Radiation
  Burns
  Chemicals
  Mechanical irritation, trauma
Drugs
  Barbiturates
  Penicillins
  Sulfonamides
  Nitrofurantoin
  Nalidixic acid
  Thiazides
  Furosemide
  Nonsteroidal anti-inflammatory agents
  Phenytoin
  Mephenytoin
  Allopurinol
  Phenolphthalein
Infections
  Bacterial
    Disseminated gonococcus, *Pseudomonas*
    Impetigo, erysipelas
    Toxic epidermal necrolysis
    Staphylococcal scalded skin syndrome
  Viral
    Herpes simplex
    Herpes zoster
    Varicella
    Variola (smallpox)
    Vaccinia
    Enterovirus (e.g., hand-foot-mouth disease)
  Syphilis, congenital
  Rickettsialpox
Erythema multiforme bullosum, Stevens-Johnson syndrome (see 10-B)
Pemphigus
Pemphigoid
Acute eczematous dermatitis, especially contact dermatitis
Dermatitis herpetiformis
Epidermolysis bullosa
Porphyria
Lupus erythematosus, discoid or systemic
Pityriasis rosea (vesicular type)
Diabetes mellitus
Herpes gestationis

Subcorneal pustular dermatosis
Bullous ichthyosis

Reference
1. Section 11: Epidermis: Disorders of Dermal and Dermal-Epidermal Cohesion—Vesicular and Bullous Disorders. In general reference 20, p 546.

11 MUSCULO-SKELETAL SYSTEM

11-A. Shoulder Pain

Fracture
Contusion
Acromial-clavicular joint separation
Rotator cuff tendinitis/impingement syndrome
Bursitis
Bicipital tendinitis (long head)
Referred pain
   Diaphragmatic irritation
      Biliary disease
      Blood or gas in peritoneal or pleural cavity
      Subphrenic abscess
      Splenic trauma
      Neoplasm
      Lower-lobe pleuropulmonary inflammatory disease
   Apical lung cancer (Pancoast syndrome)
   Cervical radiculopathy/brachial neuritis
   Angina pectoris and/or myocardial infarction
Osteoarthritis
Infectious arthritis
Rheumatoid arthritis
Crystalline arthritis
Arthritis associated with collagen-vascular disease

Shoulder-hand syndrome
Neoplasm, primary or metastatic
Local arterial, venous, or lymphatic occlusion
Adhesive capsulitis
Thoracic outlet syndromes
   Cervical and first-rib syndromes, scalenus anterior syndrome
   Hyperabduction syndrome
   Costoclavicular syndrome
Myalgias and arthralgias
Fibrositis syndromes
Psychogenic pain
Sleep dysesthesias
Congenital/developmental abnormalities
Postural

References
1. Thornhill, T: The Painful Shoulder. In general reference 21, p 435.
2. Rodnan GP, Schumacher HR (Eds): *Primer on the Rheumatic Diseases* (8th ed). Atlanta: Arthritis Foundation, 1983.
3. Bateman J: *The Shoulder and Neck*. Philadelphia: Saunders, 1978.

11-B. Back Pain

Functional, mechanical causes: Postural imbalance
    Anteroposterior (e.g., pregnancy)
    Lateral (e.g., scoliosis, unequal leg lengths)
Trauma
    Lumbar strain or sprain
    Lumbosacral disk herniation
    Vertebral fracture (compression or other)
    Subluxation of facet joints
Osteoarthritis, spondylosis
Rheumatoid arthritis
Spondylitis and/or sacroiliitis
    Ankylosing spondylitis
    Colitic (enteropathic) spondylitis
    Psoriatic arthritis
    Behçet's syndrome
    Reiter's syndrome
    Familial Mediterranean fever
    Syphilis
    Ochronosis
Spinal stenosis
    Congenital
    Degenerative
    Iatrogenic (post–laminectomy/fusion/chemonucleolysis)
    Posttraumatic
    Paget's disease
    Fluorosis
Spinal or vertebral tumor
    Benign (e.g., hemangioma, meningioma, osteoid osteoma)
    Malignant
        Primary (e.g., multiple myeloma, ependymoma, osteogenic sarcoma)
        Metastatic, especially:
            Prostate
            Non-Hodgkin's, Hodgkin's lymphoma
            Breast
            Leukemia
            Lung
            Kidney
            Thyroid
            Gastrointestinal tract
Infection (e.g., disk space infection, vertebral osteomyelitis, epidural abscess)
    Bacteria (usually secondary to hematogenous spread)
    Brucella

    Herpes zoster
    Mycobacteria
    Fungi
  Congenital causes
    Facet tropism
    Transitional vertebrae
    Spina bifida
    Spondylolysis, spondylolisthesis
  Hyperparathyroidism
  Osteomalacia (e.g., vitamin D–resistant rickets)
  Scheuermann's disease (epiphysitis)
  Radium poisoning
  Osteogenesis imperfecta
  Referred pain
    Vascular disease (especially abdominal aortic aneurysm,
        Leriche syndrome)
    Hip pain
    Pelvic or prostatic inflammation or tumor
    Retroperitoneal hematoma or tumor
    Renal disease
      Stone
      Infection
      Tumor
      Polycystic kidney disease
    Abdominal disease (e.g., intestinal, pancreatic)
    Cardiorespiratory (pulmonary emboli, pleuritis, coronary
        ischemia, pneumonitis)
Psychoneurotic causes
  Hysteria
  Malingering
  Fibrositis

References

1. Mankin HJ, Adams RD: Pain in the Back and Neck. In
   general reference 1, p 34.
2. Lipson S: Low Back Pain. In general reference 21, p 448.
3. Keim HA, Kirkaldy-Willis WH: Low Back Pain. *Clin Symp*
   32(6), 1980.

11-C. Myalgias

Fibrositis
Connective-tissue disease
  Polymyalgia rheumatica
  Rheumatoid arthritis
  Polymyositis, dermatomyositis
  Lupus erythematosus
  Polyarteritis nodosa
  Scleroderma
Systemic infection, especially:
  Viral illness
    Influenza
    Coxsackie virus infection
    Arbovirus infection
    Hepatitis
    Rabies
    Poliomyelitis
  Rheumatic fever
  Salmonellosis
  Tularemia
  Brucellosis
  Glanders
  Trichinosis
  Leptospirosis
  Relapsing fever
  Malaria
Rhabdomyolysis (see 11-D)
Drugs (e.g., amphotericin B, clofibrate, carbenoxolone)
Hypothyroidism
Hyperparathyroidism
Hypoglycemic myopathy
Congenital enzyme deficiency (e.g., phosphorylase [Mc-
    Ardle's disease], phosphofructokinase)
Polyneuropathy (e.g., Guillain-Barré disease)
Ischemic atherosclerotic disease (i.e., intermittent claudica-
    tion)

Reference
1. Part 12, Section 2: Diseases of Nerve and Muscle. In
   general reference 1, p 2047.

11-D. Muscle Weakness

*Acute or Subacute**
Electrolyte abnormality
  Hyperkalemia
  Hypokalemia
  Hypercalcemia
  Hypermagnesemia
  Hypophosphatemia
Rhabdomyolysis
  Extreme muscular exertion
  Prolonged seizures
  Hyperthermia
  Extensive crush injury or muscle infarction
  Influenza
  Hypokalemia
  Hypophosphatemia
  Alcoholic myopathy
  Snake venoms
  Industrial toxin ingestion
  Familial myoglobinuria
  Metabolic myopathies (e.g., McArdle's disease)
Polymyositis, dermatomyositis
Infection, especially:
  Viral
    Influenza
    Coxsackie virus infection
    Rabies
    Poliomyelitis
    Herpes zoster
  Trichinosis
  Toxoplasmosis
  Botulism
  Diphtheria
  Leprosy
  Cysticercosis
  Schistosomiasis
  Trypanosomiasis
  Landry-Guillain-Barré-Strohl syndrome
Peripheral neuropathy, acute (see 12-Q)
Thyrotoxicosis
Corticosteroid therapy
Organophosphorus poisoning

Chronic
Progressive muscular dystrophy, especially:
  Duchenne's

Facioscapulohumeral
Limb-girdle
Myotonic
Endocrine disorders
  Hyperthyroidism or hypothyroidism
  Hyperparathyroidism
  Vitamin D deficiency (e.g., vitamin D–deficiency rickets)
  Corticosteroid therapy
  Cushing's syndrome/Addison's disease
  Acromegaly
Connective-tissue disease
  Lupus erythematosus
  Rheumatoid arthritis
  Polymyositis, dermatomyositis
  Sjögren's syndrome
  Mixed connective-tissue disease
Alcoholic myopathy
Chronic polymyopathy
  Glycogen storage disease
  Central core disease
  McArdle's disease
  Familial periodic paralysis with progressive myopathy
Progressive neural-muscular atrophy
  Amyotrophic lateral sclerosis
  Multiple sclerosis
  Werdnig-Hoffman disease
  Peroneal muscular atrophy (Charcot-Marie-Tooth disease)
  Chronic peripheral neuropathy (e.g., arsenic, lead, nutritional) (see also 12-Q)

Intermittent and/or Transient
Electrolyte abnormality
  Hypokalemia
  Hyperkalemia
  Hypophosphatemia
  Hypercalcemia
  Hypermagnesemia
  Hyperkalemic or hypokalemic periodic paralysis
Drugs
  Aminoglycosides (especially neomycin, streptomycin, kanamycin, polymyxin B)
  Steroids
  Vincristine
  Chloroquine
  Bretylium
  Clofibrate
Myasthenia gravis

Eaton-Lambert syndrome
Acute thyrotoxic myopathy
Thyrotoxic periodic paralysis
Paramyotonia congenita
Adynamia episodica hereditaria

References
1. Part 12, Section 2: Diseases of Nerve and Muscle. In general reference 1, p 2047.
2. Bradley W: Muscle Weakness. In general reference 21, p 410.

*Developing over days to weeks. See also Intermittent and/or Transient.

11-E. Polyarticular Arthritis

Rheumatoid arthritis*
Juvenile rheumatoid arthritis*
Rheumatic fever*
Ankylosing spondylitis*
Collagen-vascular diseases
   Lupus erythematosus*
   Scleroderma*
   Polymyositis, dermatomyositis*
   Mixed connective-tissue disease
   Polyarteritis nodosa* (rare)
   Henoch-Schönlein purpura* (rare)
   Wegener's granulomatosis* (rare)
   Other vasculitides* (e.g., allergic granulomatosis) (rare)
   Polymyalgia rheumatica*
Immunologically mediated diseases
   Serum sickness*
   Hyperglobulinemic purpura*
   Hypogammaglobulinemia*
   Mixed cryoglobulinemia* (rare)
Systemic diseases
   Sjögren's syndrome*
   Reiter's syndrome*
   Psoriasis*
   Behçet's syndrome*
   Inflammatory bowel disease*
      Ulcerative colitis
      Regional enteritis
   Intestinal bypass*

Pancreatic disease
  Carcinoma
  Pancreatitis
Whipple's disease*
Familial Mediterranean fever*
Amyloidosis
Sarcoidosis*
Hematologic disorders
  Leukemia*
  Lymphoma*
  Multiple myeloma*
  Hemophilia
  Hemoglobinopathies* (especially sickle cell anemia,
    thalassemia)
Storage diseases* (e.g., Gaucher's disease, Fabry's dis-
  ease, hyperlipoproteinemia)
Ochronosis
Hemochromatosis
Wilson's disease
Acromegaly
Hypothyroidism
Renal transplantation
Degenerative joint disease
Trauma
Neuropathic arthropathy (e.g., tabes dorsalis, diabetes mel-
  litus, syringomyelia)
Joint tumor
  Pigmented villonodular synovitis
  Hemangioma
  Sarcoma
Infection*
  Bacterial (especially gonococcus, staphylococcus, pneu-
    mococcus)
  Viral (especially hepatitis B, mumps, rubella, arbovi-
    ruses)
  Tuberculous
  Fungal
  Rickettsial
  Parasitic
  Lyme disease
Others
  Gout*
  Pseudogout*
  Hypertrophic osteoarthropathy
  Intermittent hydrarthrosis*
  Palindromic rheumatism*
  Radiation
  Relapsing polychondritis*

Acute tropical polyarthritis*
Tietze's syndrome
Nonarticular rheumatism
Bursitis*
Periarthritis*
Tendinitis*
Tenosynovitis*
Epicondylitis
Myositis
Fibrositis
Fasciitis

References

1. General reference 21.
2. Bennett JC: Infectious Etiology of Rheumatoid Arthritis. *Arthritis Rheum* 21:531, 1978.

*Usually inflammatory (i.e., joints painful, swollen, stiff, often erythematous and warm).

11-F. Monoarticular (or Oligoarticular) Arthritis

Juvenile rheumatoid arthritis
Ankylosing spondylitis
Rheumatoid arthritis (rare)
Systemic diseases
Psoriasis
Behçet's syndrome
Inflammatory bowel disease (ulcerative colitis, regional enteritis)
Pancreatic disease (carcinoma, pancreatitis)

Whipple's disease
Familial Mediterranean fever
Hematologic disorders
    Leukemia
    Lymphoma
    Bleeding-clotting disorders (hemophilia, von Wille-
      brand's disease, anticoagulant use)
    Hemoglobinopathies (especially sickle cell anemia,
      thalassemia)
Storage diseases (e.g., Gaucher's, Fabry's)
Acromegaly
Amyloidosis
Degenerative joint disease
Trauma
Neuropathic arthropathy (e.g., tabes dorsalis, diabetes mel-
  litus, syringomyelia)
Joint tumors (e.g., pigmented villonodular synovitis, he-
  mangioma, sarcoma)
Infection
    Bacterial (especially gonococcus, staphylococcus, pneu-
      mococcus)
    Viral (especially hepatitis B, rubella, mumps)
    Tuberculous
    Fungal
    Rickettsial
    Parasitic
Others
    Gout
    Pseudogout
    Intermittent hydrarthrosis
    Loose joint body
    Foreign body
    Palindromic rheumatism
    Radiation
    Relapsing polychondritis
Nonarticular rheumatism
    Bursitis
    Periarthritis
    Tendinitis
    Tenosynovitis
    Epicondylitis
    Myositis
    Fibrositis
    Fasciitis

Reference

1. Schmid F: Approach to Monoarticular Arthritis. In general
   reference 21, p 391.

11-G. Characteristics of Synovial Fluid

	Normal	Noninflammatory	Inflammatory	Purulent	Hemorrhagic
Color	Clear to pale yellow	Xanthochromic	Xanthochromic to white	White	
Clarity	Transparent	Transparent	Translucent to opaque	Opaque	
Viscosity	High	High	Low	Low*	
Mucin clot	Good	Good to fair	Fair to poor	Poor	
Spontaneous clot	None	Often	Often	Often	
WBCs/mm^3	<150	<3000	3000–50,000	>50,000	
% Polymorphs	<25	<25	>70	>90	
Glucose (mg/dl)	Nearly equal to blood	Nearly equal to blood	>25, lower than blood	>50, lower than blood	
Culture	**Negative**	**Negative**	**Negative**	**Often positive**	

| Conditions in which findings are likely to occur | Osteoarthritis Trauma Neuropathic arthropathy SLE Acute rheumatic fever Pigmented villonodular synovitis Erythema nodosum Polyarteritis nodosa Amyloidosis | Rheumatoid arthritis Connective tissue diseases (SLE, PSS, DM/PM) Viral arthritis Ankylosing spondylitis Acute gout or pseudogout Seronegative spondyloarthropathies (Reiter's syndrome, psoriatic arthritis, inflammatory bowel disease arthritis) | Bacterial arthritis | Trauma Anticoagulation Neuropathic arthropathy: Charcot joints Joint tumor Hematologic disorders (especially hemophilia, sickle cell trait or disease) |

Key: SLE = systemic lupus erythematosus; PSS = progressive systemic sclerosis; DM/PM = dermatomyositis/polymyositis.
*May be high in infection with coagulase-positive staphylococcus.
Source: Group designations from Ropes MW, Bauer W: *Synovial Fluid Changes in Joint Diseases.* Cambridge, Mass.: Harvard University Press, 1953. Table modified from McCarty DJ: Synovial Fluid. In McCarty DJ (Ed): *Arthritis and Allied Conditions* (9th ed.). Philadelphia: Lea & Febiger, 1979, pp 52–56. Copyright © 1979 by Lea & Febiger; and Rodnan GP, Schumacher HR (Eds): *Primer on Rheumatic Diseases* (8th ed.) Atlanta, GA: Arthritis Foundation, 1983, p 187.

11-H. Clubbing

Usually with Hypertrophic Osteoarthropathy
Neoplasm
  Intrathoracic
    Lung
    Pleura
    Mediastinum (Hodgkin's disease)
    Thymus
  Esophagus, stomach
  Intestine
  Liver
Other pulmonary disorders
  Lung abscess
  Empyema
  Chronic pneumonitis
  Pneumoconiosis
  Bronchiectasis
  Tuberculosis
  Cystic fibrosis
Idiopathic, hereditary (pachydermoperiostitis)

Usually Without Hypertrophic Osteoarthropathy
Genetic
Subacute bacterial endocarditis
Cyanotic congenital heart disease
Chronic liver disease (e.g., biliary cirrhosis)
Intestinal disorders
  Ulcerative colitis
  Regional enteritis
  Sprue, steatorrhea
  Bacterial or amebic dysentery
  Tuberculosis, intestinal
Hyperparathyroidism
Graves' disease (thyroid acropathy)
Occupational trauma (e.g., jackhammer operation)

Unilateral
Aneurysm of aorta or of subclavian, innominate, or brachial
    artery
Shoulder subluxation
Hemiplegia
Axillary or apical lung tumor

Unidigital
Median nerve injury

Sarcoidosis
Tophaceous gout

Reference
1. Altman RD, Tenenbaum J: Hypertrophic Osteoarthropathy. In general reference 21, p 1594.

11-I. Raynaud's Phenomenon

Raynaud's disease
Chronic arterial disease
    Atherosclerosis
    Thromboangiitis obliterans
    Thrombosis
    Embolism
Pulmonary veno-occlusive disease
Collagen-vascular disease
    Scleroderma
    Lupus erythematosus
    Rheumatoid arthritis
    Polyarteritis nodosa
    Mixed connective-tissue disease
    Polymyositis, dermatomyositis
    Sjögren's syndrome
Occupational exposure
    Vibration (e.g., pneumatic tools)
    Percussion (e.g., typing)
    Vinyl chloride polymerization
Drugs, toxins
    Heavy metals (lead, arsenic, thallium)
    Methysergide, ergot compounds
    Propranolol
Hematologic disorders
    Dysproteinemias (e.g., multiple myeloma, Waldenström's macroglobulinemia)
    Polycythemia vera
    Leukemia
    Cryoglobulinemia
    Cold agglutinin phenomenon
Neurologic disorders
    Peripheral neuropathy
    Hemiplegia
    Intervertebral disk herniation

Spinal cord tumor
Multiple sclerosis
Transverse myelitis
Syringomyelia
Carpal tunnel syndrome
Thoracic outlet syndrome
Posttraumatic reflex sympathetic dystrophy
Post-cold injury (e.g., frostbite)
Acromegaly
Myxedema
Fabry's disease

References
1. General reference 1.
2. Spittell JA: Raynaud's Phenomenon and Allied Vaso-spastic Conditions. In Fairbairn JF, Juergens JL, Spittell JA (Eds): *Allen-Barker-Hines Peripheral Vascular Diseases* (4th ed). Philadelphia: Saunders, 1972, p 387.

11-J. Osteomalacia

Vitamin D deficiency
    Dietary deficiency
    Insufficient sun exposure
    Malabsorption (e.g., pancreatic insufficiency, small-intestine disease, postgastrectomy)
Disordered vitamin D metabolism (hereditary or acquired)
    Chronic renal failure
    Anticonvulsant therapy
    Chronic liver disease (e.g., biliary cirrhosis)
Chronic acidosis (e.g., distal renal tubular acidosis, chronic acetazolamide ingestion, ureterosigmoidostomy)
Phosphate depletion (see 1-O)
Impaired renal tubular phosphate resorption
    Vitamin D–resistant rickets
    Fanconi syndrome (hereditary or acquired)
    Tumor phosphaturia
    Neurofibromatosis
    Neonatal (transient)
    Intoxications (cadmium, lead, outdated tetracycline)
Miscellaneous
    Osteopetrosis
    Hypophosphatasia
    Fluorosis

Magnesium-dependent conditions
Parenteral hyperalimentation

References

1. Dent CE, Stamp TCB: Vitamin D, Rickets, and Osteomalacia. In Avioli LV, Krane SM (Eds): *Metabolic Bone Disease.* New York: Academic, 1977, p 237.
2. Krane SM, Holick MF: Metabolic Bone Disease. In general reference 1, p 1889.

11-K. Osteopenia*

Aging (especially postmenopause)†
Immobilization
Nutritional causes
  Calcium and/or vitamin D deficiency
  Malnutrition, malabsorption
  Postgastrectomy
  Scurvy
Corticosteroid excess
  Cushing's syndrome or disease
  Steroid therapy
Other endocrine disorders
  Hypogonadism (e.g., Klinefelter's syndrome, Turner's
    syndrome, early oophorectomy)
  Thyrotoxicosis
  Acromegaly
  Hyperparathyroidism
  Hypopituitarism
  Diabetes mellitus
Inherited connective-tissue diseases
  Homocystinuria
  Marfan's syndrome
  Ehlers-Danlos syndrome
  Osteogenesis imperfecta
Rheumatoid arthritis
Ankylosing spondylitis
Malignancy, especially:
  Lymphoma
  Leukemia
  Multiple myeloma
  Waldenström's macroglobulinemia
  Systemic mastocytosis
  Carcinomatosis

Heparin therapy (chronic)†
Chronic obstructive pulmonary disease†
Chronic acidosis (especially renal tubular acidosis, metabolic acidosis secondary to high-protein diet)
Alcoholism
Hepatic insufficiency, cirrhosis (alcoholic or other)
Methotrexate†
Epilepsy
Chronic renal failure (renal osteodystrophy)
Paget's disease (with predominantly lytic lesions)
Juvenile (idiopathic)†
Cystic fibrosis†
Riley-Day syndrome
Menkes' syndrome
Down's syndrome
Hypophosphatasia, adult variety
Female distance runners
Smoking

References

1. Avioli LV: Osteoporosis: Pathogenesis and Therapy. In Avioli LV, Krane SM (Eds): *Metabolic Bone Disease.* New York: Academic, 1977, p 307.
2. Riggs BL, Melton LJ: Involutional Osteoporosis. *N Engl J Med* 314:26, 1986.

*Decreased bone mass.
†Characterized on bone biopsy by decreased bone mass with normal mineral-to-matrix ratio.

11-L. Antibodies to Nuclear or Cytoplasmic Antigens

Disease	Antibodies most commonly associated
Systemic lupus erythematosus	Anti-native (double-stranded) DNA
	Anti-single-stranded DNA
	Anti-ribonucleoprotein (anti-RNP)
	Anti-Sm
	Anti-Ro/SSA
	Anti-La/SSB
	Anti-histone (especially with drug-induced lupus)
Progressive systemic sclerosis	Antinucleolar
	Anticentromere
	Anti-Scl-70 (especially in scleroderma/polymyositis overlap syndrome)
	Anti-RNP
Polymyositis	Anti-Jo$_1$
	Anti-Scl-70
Mixed connective tissue disease	Anti-RNP
Sjögren's syndrome	Anti-Ro/SSA
	Anti-La/SSB

References
1. General reference 21.
2. Rodnan GP, Schumacher HR (Eds): *Primer on the Rheumatic Diseases* (8th ed). Atlanta: Arthritis Foundation, 1983, p 56.
3. Reichlin M: Significance of Ro Antigen System. *J Clin Immunol* 6(5):339, 1986.

11-M. Rheumatoid Factor

Aging
Rheumatoid arthritis
Systemic lupus erythematosus
Scleroderma
Dermatomyositis, polymyositis
Infections
   Syphilis
   Influenza
   Subacute bacterial endocarditis
   Infectious mononucleosis
   Bacterial bronchitis
   Viral hepatitis
   Tuberculosis
   Leprosy
   Parasitic infection (e.g., schistosomiasis, kala azar)
   Following extensive immunizations
Sjögren's syndrome (with or without arthritis)
Chronic active hepatitis and cirrhosis
Lymphoma
Waldenström's macroglobulinemia
Mixed cryoglobulinemia
Hyperglobulinemic purpura
Chronic lung disease
   Pneumoconioses (e.g., silicosis, asbestosis)
   Sarcoidosis
   Interstitial fibrosis, idiopathic
Multiple transfusions
Renal transplantation

Reference
1. Lipsky PE: Rheumatoid Arthritis. In general reference 1, p 1423.

11-N. Systemic Lupus Erythematosus Criteria*

Facial erythema (butterfly rash)
Discoid lupus erythematosus
Photosensitivity
Nonerosive arthritis
Oral or nasopharyngeal ulceration
Serositis (pleuritis and/or pericarditis)
Psychosis and/or seizures
Proteinuria > 0.5 gm/day or cellular casts in urine (red cell, hemoglobin, granular, tubular, mixed)
Hematologic disorder:
  Hemolytic anemia, leukopenia (WBC < 4000/mm^3), lymphopenia (< 1500/mm^3), or thrombocytopenia (< 100,000/mm^3)
Antinuclear antibody
Immunologic disorder: positive LE cell preparation, anti-DNA antibodies, anti-Sm antibodies. or chronic false-positive serologic test for syphilis

*From Tan EM, Cohen AS, Fries JF, et al: The 1982 Revised Criteria for the Classification of Systemic Lupus Erythematosus (SLE). *Arthritis Rheum* 25:1271, 1982. Diagnosis of systemic lupus can be made if 4 or more of the above 11 criteria are present, serially or simultaneously, during any interval of observation.

12 NERVOUS SYSTEM

12-A. Dizziness and Vertigo

Dizziness
Hyperventilation
Anxiety, psychosomatic causes
Hypoxia
Anemia
Hypotension (especially orthostatic)
Hypertension

True Vertigo
Infection
    Labyrinthitis (bacterial, viral, syphilitic)
    Cholesteatoma
    Chronic otitis media with middle-ear fistula
    Vestibular neuritis/neuropathy
    Herpes zoster oticus
Vascular disorders
    Vertebrobasilar insufficiency or occlusion
    Labyrinthine or internal auditory artery occlusion or
        spasm
    Migraine

Hemorrhage into labyrinthine system, brainstem, or cere-
bellum (e.g., secondary to bleeding diathesis, leuke-
mia, hypertension)
Ménière's disease
Benign positional vertigo of Bárány
Drugs and toxins
    Alcohol
    Quinine
    Aminoglycoside antibiotics (especially streptomycin, gen-
        tamicin)
    Salicylates
    Benzene
    Arsenic
    Arsine
Trauma
    Temporal bone fracture
    Labyrinthine concussion
    Postsurgical (inner-ear area)
Tumor, especially:
    Acoustic neuroma
    Epidermoid carcinoma
    Metastatic carcinoma (especially breast, kidney, lung,
        stomach)
    Glomus body tumor
Other
    Extraocular muscle palsy
    Motion sickness
    Multiple sclerosis
    Syringobulbia
    Tabes dorsalis
    Friedreich's ataxia
    Encephalitis
    Seizure aura

References

1. Haymaker W, Kuhlenbeck H: Disorders of the Brainstem
   and Its Cranial Nerves. In general reference 23, vol 3,
   chap 40.
2. Baloh RW: Neurotology. In general reference 23, vol 3,
   chap 42.
3. General reference 22, p 211.

12-B. Headache

Muscle contraction (tension)
Migraine (including cluster headache)
Nonmigrainous vascular causes
  Effort (physical activity)
  Vasomotor rhinitis
  Fever
  Hypertension
  Hypotension
  Hypoxia (e.g., chronic obstructive pulmonary disease,
    pulmonary infiltrative disease, sleep apnea syn-
    drome, altitude)
  Anemia
  Cerebrovascular disease (thrombosis, embolism, hemor-
    rhage)
  Postseizure
  Endocrine causes
    Hypoglycemia
    Hypothyroidism
    Hyperthyroidism
    Adrenal insufficiency
Drugs and toxins
  Theophylline
  Caffeine and caffeine withdrawal
  Nitrates
  Nitrites (e.g., hot dogs)
  Dextroamphetamines
  Ephedrine
  Reserpine
  Monamine oxidase inhibitors + catecholamines
  Histamine
  Steroid withdrawal
  Alcohol withdrawal
  Disulfiram (Antabuse) + alcohol
  Lead
  Benzene
  Carbon monoxide
  Carbon tetrachloride
  Insecticides
Intracranial causes
  Tumor
  Arteriovenous malformation
  Aneurysm (with or without hemorrhage)
  Subdural hematoma
  Encephalitis, brain abscess
  Pseudotumor

Posttraumatic
Cranial inflammation
  Meningeal irritation
    Infection, especially tuberculous or fungal
    Carcinomatous infiltration
  Postsubarachnoid hemorrhage
  Vasculitis (e.g., temporal arteritis, lupus, polyarteritis nodosa)
Cranial and neck causes
  Sinuses (trauma, inflammation)
  Ears (external, middle, internal)
  Eyes (inflammation, trauma, increased intraocular pressure, poor refraction)
  Teeth, jaws (infection, trauma, temporomandibular joint malocclusion)
  Cervical spine, ligaments, muscles (trauma, cervical spondylosis, ankylosing spondylitis, tumor)
Psychogenic, psychiatric

References
1. Friedman AP: Headache. In general reference 23, vol 2, chap 13.
2. General reference 22, p 129.

12-C. Paresthesias

Peripheral neuropathy (see 12-Q), especially associated
    with:
  Diabetes mellitus
  Alcoholism
  Thiamine deficiency
Peripheral nerve entrapment, compression, trauma (e.g.,
    intervertebral disk herniation, thoracic duct outlet syn-
    drome, carpal tunnel syndrome)
Atherosclerotic peripheral vascular disease
Spinal cord disease
  Spinal cord or nerve root compression
  Multiple sclerosis
  Tabes dorsalis
  Subacute combined degeneration of spinal cord (perni-
    cious anemia, vitamin B_{12} deficiency)
  Strachan's syndrome
Metabolic disturbance
  Hypocalcemia
  Respiratory alkalosis

References
1. General reference 1.
2. General reference 22.

12-D. Syncope

Neurological and/or Mechanical Causes
Mediated by vagal stimulation and/or autonomic insufficiency
- Vasovagal reaction (often associated with strong emotion or pain)
- Prolonged recumbency or inactivity
- Peripheral neuropathy with autonomic involvement (e.g., diabetes, amyloidosis, tabes dorsalis)
- Drugs (e.g., nitrates, antihypertensive agents, ganglionic blockers, alcohol)
- Carotid sinus syncope
- Micturition syncope
- Swallow syncope
- Bowel stimulation/defecation syncope
- Airway stimulation
- Eyeball pressure
- Glossopharyngeal neuralgia
- Sympathectomy
- Primary autonomic insufficiency
Seizure
Head trauma
Reduced cardiac output/venous return
- Hypovolemia
- Hypotension
- Valsalva maneuver
  - Cough
  - Voluntary forced expiration against closed glottis
  - Weight lifting
- Atrial myxoma or thrombus
- Cardiac tamponade

Cardiopulmonary Causes
Cardiac arrhythmias (see 2-O)
- Bradyarrhythmias (e.g., sick sinus syndrome)
- Tachyarrhythmias (especially ventricular fibrillation, ventricular tachycardia, paroxysmal atrial tachycardia)
- Atrioventricular block
Pulmonary embolism
Myocardial infarction with cardiogenic shock
Pericardial tamponade
Aortic stenosis
Pulmonic stenosis
Primary pulmonary hypertension

Cerebrovascular Causes
Atherosclerotic disease of carotid and/or cerebral vessels
(especially vertebral-basilar insufficiency)
Takayasu's disease
Hypertensive encephalopathy
Cervical spine abnormalities (e.g., cervical spondylosis)

Metabolic Causes
Anemia
Hypoxia
Hyperventilation
Hypoglycemia

Psychological Causes
Anxiety, hysteria

References
1. General reference 22, p 273.
2. Johnson RJ, Lambie DG, Spalding JMK: The Autonomic
Nervous System. In general reference 23, vol 4, chap 57.

12-E. Deafness

Sensorineural (Inner Ear)
Aging
Prolonged exposure to loud noise
Drugs
   Salicylates
   Aminoglycoside antibiotics (especially neomycin, amika-
      cin)
   Furosemide, ethacrynic acid
   Quinine
Infection
   Chronic middle or inner ear infection
   Cholesteatoma
   Labyrinthitis
      Bacterial
      Viral (e.g., mumps)
      Syphilis (usually congenital)
   Herpes zoster oticus
Ménière's disease
Tumor of eighth nerve or cerebellopontine angle (especially
     acoustic neuroma)
Eighth nerve infarction
Multiple sclerosis
Hereditary or congenital causes (e.g., congenital rubella,
     Alport's syndrome)

Conductive
Cerumen impaction
Otosclerosis
Chronic otitis media, cholesteatoma
Trauma (including temporal bone fracture, bleeding into
     middle ear)
Mucopolysaccharidoses

References
1. General reference 22, p 211.
2. Baloh RW: Neurotology. In general reference 23, vol 3,
   chap 42.

12-F. Ataxia

Cerebellar Disease (Cerebellar Ataxia)
Alcoholic cerebellar degeneration, Wernicke's disease
Degenerative or demyelinating diseases (e.g., multiple
    sclerosis, Huntington's chorea, Creutzfeldt-Jakob dis-
    ease)
Neoplasm
Vascular occlusion (basilar artery or its branches)
Vasculitis (e.g., systemic lupus erythematosus, polyarteritis
    nodosa)
Encephalitis
Brain abscess
Cranial trauma
Posthyperthermia, heat stroke
Hypoxic encephalopathy
Drugs (e.g., phenytoin, barbiturates)
Toxins (e.g., arsenic, lead, mercury)
Nonwilsonian hepatocerebral degeneration (posthepatic
    coma)
Hypoparathyroidism
Congenital
Hereditary diseases (e.g., phenylketonuria, ataxia-telan-
    giectasia, metachromatic leukodystrophy, abetalipopro-
    teinemia)
Primary cerebellar ataxias (e.g., olivopontocerebellar atro-
    phy, dentate cerebellar ataxia)

Loss of Postural or Proprioceptive Sense (Sensory Ataxia)
Infection (e.g., neurosyphilis)
Endocrine disease (e.g., diabetes mellitus)
Toxins (e.g., arsenic, ergot)
Nutritional diseases
    Alcoholism
    Beriberi
    Pellagra
    Vitamin B_{12} deficiency
    Scurvy
Hereditary disease (e.g., Friedreich's ataxia)
Congenital
Other
    Multiple sclerosis
    Amyotrophic lateral sclerosis
    Primary posterolateral sclerosis
    Spinal cord tumor or compression

References
1. Brown JR: Diseases of the Cerebellum. In general reference 23, vol 3, chap 37.
2. General reference 22.

12-G. Acute Confusional State*

Delirium†
Drug withdrawal after chronic intoxication, especially:
   Alcohol
   Barbiturates
   Other sedatives
Drug intoxication, especially:
   Atropine
   Amphetamines
   Bromides
   Caffeine
   Camphor
   Ergot
   Scopolamine
Infectious and febrile illness, especially:
   Septicemia
   Pneumonia
   Typhoid fever
   Rheumatic fever
Central nervous system disorders
   Cerebrovascular disease (especially involving parietal or temporal lobes or upper brainstem)
   Brain tumor
   Encephalitis (especially viral)
   Meningitis
   Subarachnoid hemorrhage
   Head trauma (e.g., concussion, subdural hematoma)
   Postseizures
Thyrotoxicosis
Steroid psychosis (rare)

Other Acute Confusional States‡
Metabolic causes
  Electrolyte disorders, especially:
    Hyponatremia
    Hypercalcemia
    Hypokalemia
  Hypoxia
  Hypercarbia
  Congestive heart failure
  Hypoglycemia
  Hepatic encephalopathy
  Uremia
  Hypothyroidism
  Wernicke's disease
  Porphyria
Drug intoxication
  Barbiturates
  Narcotics
  Bromides
  Antihypertensive agents
Central nervous system disease
  Cerebrovascular disease (see 12-N)
  Brain tumor
  Brain abscess
  Meningitis
  Encephalitis
  Migraine
  Subdural or epidural hematoma
Febrile illness
Acute psychosis (e.g., postoperative, postpartum)
Preexisting dementia with superimposed stress (e.g., Alzheimer's, serious illness) (see 12-H)

Reference
1. General reference 22, p 301.

*See also 12-H and 12-M.
†An acute, transient confusional state characterized by mental alertness, gross disorientation, hallucinations, psychomotor and autonomic hyperactivity.
‡Confusional states not associated with psychomotor or autonomic hyperactivity.

12-H. Dementia*

Degenerative diseases
  Senile dementia
  Alzheimer's disease
  Cerebral arteriosclerosis, multiple cerebrovascular accidents
  Pick's disease (circumscribed cerebral atrophy)
  Parkinson's disease
  Korsakoff's psychosis
  Demyelinating disease (e.g., multiple sclerosis, Schilder's disease [diffuse cerebral sclerosis])
  Amyotrophic lateral sclerosis
  Progressive supranuclear palsy (Steele-Richardson-Olszewski syndrome)
Metabolic causes
  Hypoxic encephalopathy
  Hypoglycemia
  Hypocalcemia (e.g., hypoparathyroidism)
  Hepatocerebral degeneration (posthepatic coma)
  Pernicious anemia, subacute combined degeneration of the spinal cord
  Pellagra
  Myxedema
  Cushing's disease
  Barbiturate intoxication, chronic
  Bromide intoxication
  Dialysis dementia
Infectious causes
  Brain abscess
  Chronic meningoencephalitis (e.g., cryptococcosis, neurosyphilis)
  Viral encephalitis (especially herpes simplex)
  Acquired immunodeficiency syndrome (AIDS)
  Progressive multifocal leukoencephalopathy
  Creutzfeldt-Jakob disease
Intracranial tumor
Head trauma (e.g., contusion, hemorrhage, subdural hematoma)
Myoclonic epilepsy
Normal-pressure hydrocephalus
Hereditary diseases
  Huntington's chorea
  Wilson's disease
  Lipid storage diseases (e.g., Tay-Sachs, leukodystrophies)
  Mucopolysaccharidoses

Pseudodementias
    Depression
    Hypomania
    Schizophrenia
    Hysteria

Reference
1. General reference 22, p 311.

*Deterioration of intellectual and cognitive functions with little or no
disturbance of consciousness or perception. See also 12-G and 12-
M.

12-I. Tremor

Tremor at rest (present at rest, decreased with movement)
    Parkinson's disease
    Postencephalitic parkinsonism
    Wilson's disease
    Phenothiazines (tardive dyskinesia)
    Brain tumor
Action tremor (present with movement, decreased at rest)
    Physiologic (anxiety, fatigue)
    Essential (senile and/or familial)
    Withdrawal from alcohol or opiates
    Meningoencephalitis (e.g., viral, paretic neurosyphilis)
    Hyperthyroidism
    Pheochromocytoma
    Carcinoid syndrome
    Bronchodilators, beta agonists
    Xanthines (e.g., coffee, tea)
    Steroids
    Lithium
Ataxic (increased at terminal phase of voluntary movement)
        (see 12-F)

Reference
1. General reference 22, p 76.

12-J. Choreoathetosis

Hereditary diseases, especially:
  Wilson's disease
  Huntington's disease
  Lesch-Nyhan disease
  Lipid storage disease (e.g., Niemann-Pick)
  Dystonia musculorum deformans
Drugs
  Phenothiazines
  Haloperidol
  L-Dopa
  Dihydroxyphenylalanine
  Bromocriptine
Postinfectious (Sydenham's chorea)
  Rheumatic fever
  Diphtheria
  Rubella
  Pertussis
Pregnancy (chorea gravidarum)
Hypoxic encephalopathy
Kernicterus
Perinatal hypoxia or injury
Hyperthyroidism
Nonwilsonian hepatocerebral degeneration (posthepatic
  coma)
Lupus erythematosus
Acute disseminated encephalomyelitis (postinfectious,
  postvaccinal)
Corticostriatospinal degeneration
Thalamic infarct or hemorrhage

References
1. McDowell FH, Lee JE, Sweet RD: Extrapyramidal Disease. In general reference 23, vol 3, chap 38.
2. General reference 22.

12-K. Nystagmus

Pendular*
Congenital
Spasmus nutans
Associated with bilateral central loss of vision before 2
  years of age
 Albinism
 Aniridia
 Bilateral chorioretinitis
 Congenital cataracts
 Corneal scarring
 Optic atrophy
Multiple sclerosis
Prolonged work in dim light (miner's nystagmus)

Jerk†
Nonpathologic
 Extreme lateral gaze
 Attempt to fix on moving objects (opticokinetic nystag-
  mus)
 Labyrinthine stimulation (e.g., cold water in auditory
  canal)
Drugs
 Barbiturates
 Alcohol
 Phenytoin
 Phenothiazines
 Meperidine
Labyrinthine-vestibular disease (see 12-A)
Cerebellar lesions (e.g., Wernicke's disease, cerebellopon-
  tine angle tumor)
Encephalitis
Vascular disease involving brainstem (especially hyperten-
  sive infarction, posterior inferior cerebellar artery occlu-
  sion)
Demyelinating disease (e.g., multiple sclerosis)
Brainstem tumor
Syringobulbia
Meningioma, meningeal cyst
Arnold-Chiari malformation
Congenital

Reference
1. General reference 22, p 194.
*Both components equal.
†Fast and slow components.

12-L. Seizures

Central Nervous System and Vascular Causes
Cerebrovascular disease (see 12-N)
  Thrombosis
  Embolism
  Hemorrhage (intracerebral or subarachnoid)
  Vasculitis (especially lupus erythematosus, polyarteritis
      nodosa, mixed connective tissue disease)
  Infarction
  Thrombophlebitis
  Arteriovenous malformation
Brain tumor (especially metastatic tumor, meningioma, as-
    trocytoma)
Cerebral infection
  Encephalitis
  Meningitis (especially bacterial)
  Brain abscess
  Neurosyphilis
  Creutzfeldt-Jakob disease
Head trauma
Hypoxic encephalopathy
Reduced cerebral blood flow (e.g., hypotension, Stokes-
    Adams syndrome, carotid sinus syncope)
Hypertensive encephalopathy
Eclampsia
Alzheimer's disease
Pick's disease

Metabolic Causes
Fever
Alcohol withdrawal
Barbiturate withdrawal
Drugs, toxins
  Amphetamines
  Heroin
  Cocaine
  Phenothiazines
  Tricyclic antidepressants
  Lidocaine
  Aminophylline
  Salicylates
  Ergot
  Digitalis
  Penicillins
  Nalidixic acid

Isoniazid
Cycloserine
Physostigmine, other anticholinergics
Vincristine
Lithium
Lead
Mercury
Arsenic
Thallium
Strychnine
Camphor
Hypoglycemia
Hyperglycemia
Hyponatremia
Hypernatremia (or rapid correction of hypernatremia)
Hypocalcemia
Hypomagnesemia
Alkalosis (respiratory or metabolic)
Uremia
Dialysis dysequilibrium
Hepatic failure
Reye's syndrome
Thyrotoxicosis
Hypothyroidism
Pyridoxine deficiency
Pellagra

Congenital or Inherited Diseases
Congenital infection
 Toxoplasmosis
 Cytomegalovirus
 Syphilis
 Rubella (maternal)
Neonatal hypoxia or trauma, kernicterus
Down's syndrome
Lipid storage disease (e.g., Gaucher's disease)
Tuberous sclerosis
Sturge-Weber disease
Phenylketonuria
Acute intermittent porphyria

Idiopathic

References
1. General reference 22, p 233.
2. Forster FM, Booker HE: The Epilepsies and Convulsive
   Disorders. In general reference 23, vol 3, chap 31.

12-M. Coma*

Primary neurologic disease
    Cerebrovascular accident (thrombosis, embolism, hemor-
        rhage—see 12-N), especially involving upper brain-
        stem
    Hypertensive encephalopathy
    Head trauma
    Intracranial neoplasm
    Seizures and postictal state
    Meningitis, encephalitis, brain abscess
    Other
        Demyelinating disease (e.g., multiple sclerosis, central
            pontine myelinolysis, Schilder's disease)
        Creutzfeldt-Jakob disease
        Progressive multifocal leukoencephalopathy
        Marchiafava-Bignami disease
Metabolic causes
    Drugs, especially:
        Barbiturates
        Benzodiazepines
        Anesthetics
        Phenothiazines
        Narcotics
        Alcohol
    Toxins (e.g., methanol, carbon monoxide)
    Hypoxia
    Hypercapnia
    Shock (e.g., septic, cardiogenic) (see 2-K)
    Acidosis, metabolic or respiratory (e.g., diabetic ketoaci-
        dosis)
    Hyperthermia or hypothermia
    Hypernatremia or hyponatremia
    Hypercalcemia
    Hypoglycemia
    Hepatic failure
    Reye's syndrome
    Uremia (also dialysis dysequilibrium, dialysis dementia)
    Pancreatitis, acute
    Myxedema
    Thyrotoxicosis
    Adrenal insufficiency
    Thiamine deficiency
Hysteria

References
1. General reference 22, p 255.
2. Plum F, Posner JB: *Diagnosis of Stupor and Coma* (3rd ed). Philadelphia: Davis, 1980.

*See also 12-G and 12-H.

12-N. Cerebrovascular Disease

Thrombosis and/or Vascular Occlusion
Thrombosis, atherosclerotic
Hypotension in presence of atherosclerotic carotid disease
    (e.g., hypovolemia, Stokes-Adams attack, myocardial
    infarction)
Vasculitis (especially arteritis)
  Infectious
    Subacute bacterial meningitis
    Meningovascular syphilis
    Tuberculous meningitis
    Fungal meningitis
    Protozoan and parasitic meningitis (e.g., malaria, tri-
      chinosis, schistosomiasis)
  Noninfectious
    Systemic lupus erythematosus
    Polyarteritis nodosa
    Necrotizing arteritis
    Granulomatous arteritis
    Temporal arteritis
    Takayasu's disease
Cerebral thrombophlebitis and/or venous sinus thrombosis

(usually associated with infection of ear, sinus, face, or meninges)
Oral contraceptives
Hematologic disorders
  Sickle cell disease
  Polycythemia vera
  Thrombotic thrombocytopenic purpura
  Hyperproteinemic or hyperviscosity states
Carotid artery trauma
Radiation
Dissecting aneurysm of carotid artery (e.g., secondary to cystic medial necrosis or dissecting aortic aneurysm)
Pressure secondary to intracerebral hematoma
Migraine syndrome
Fibromuscular dysplasia
Fabry's disease
Homocystinuria
Moyamoya disease

Embolism
Atrial arrhythmias (especially atrial fibrillation—usually with rheumatic valvular or atherosclerotic cardiovascular disease)
Rheumatic heart disease, especially mitral stenosis (with or without atrial fibrillation)
Myocardial infarction with mural thrombus
Cardiac surgery, complications of (e.g., air, platelet, fat, silicone embolism)
Prosthetic heart valve
Endocarditis
  Bacterial
  Nonbacterial (e.g., associated with carcinomatosis or systemic lupus erythematosus)
Atherosclerotic embolism from other arteries
  Aorta or carotid arteries (e.g., secondary to carotid massage or arteriography)
  Vertebral or basilar arteries
Pulmonary vein thrombosis (especially septic or tumor emboli)
Fat embolism
Tumor embolism
Air embolism
Venous thromboembolism with cardiac or pulmonary right-to-left shunt (paradoxic embolism)
Atrial myxoma
Trichinosis

Hemorrhage

Hypertension (including hypertensive encephalopathy)
Aneurysm (ruptured or unruptured)
  Saccular ("berry")
  Fusiform (atherosclerotic)
  Mycotic
Arteriovenous malformation, ruptured or unruptured
Hemorrhagic disorders (e.g., thrombocytopenia, thrombo-
    cytosis, coagulopathy, disseminated intravascular co-
    agulation, anticoagulant therapy)
Intracranial trauma (e.g., acute extradural or subdural he-
    matoma, intracerebral hemorrhage)
Hemorrhage into tumor
Hemorrhagic infarction
Connective-tissue disease (especially lupus erythematosus
    and polyarteritis nodosa)

Reference

1. General reference 22, p 569.

12-O. Paralysis (or Paresis)*

Acute (Developing in Hours)

Spinal cord injury
Spinal cord hemorrhage (secondary to vascular malforma-
    tion, coagulopathy, anticoagulant therapy, trauma)
Spinal cord infarct (secondary to spinal artery thrombosis,
    embolism, vasculitis)
Dissecting aortic aneurysm
Aortic thrombosis
Acute necrotizing myelitis
Profound hypokalemia (serum K^+ < 2.5 mEq/L)†
Hyperkalemic or hypokalemic periodic paralysis†
Hypermagnesemia†

Subacute (Developing in Days)

Guillain-Barré syndrome
Myelitis
  Viral (especially polio, rabies, herpes zoster)
  Postinfectious (especially after measles, smallpox, chick-
    enpox)
  Postvaccinal (especially after rabies or smallpox vaccina-
    tion)
  Subacute pyogenic meningomyelitis

Tuberculous meningomyelitis
Acute demyelinating myelitis (e.g., multiple sclerosis)
Acute necrotizing myelitis
Rhabdomyolysis
Crush injury
Excessive muscular activity
Muscle infarction secondary to prolonged pressure and
ischemia
Polymyositis, viral or idiopathic
Diphtheritic polyneuropathy
Botulism‡
Spinal cord or epidural abscess
Spinal cord compression (e.g., secondary to tumor)

Slow (Developing over Weeks to Months)
Severe peripheral neuropathy (see 12-Q)
Multiple cerebrovascular accidents (bilateral hemiplegia)†
Polymyositis
    Infection-associated
        Viral infection
        Syphilis
        Tuberculosis
        Toxoplasmosis, other protozoan or fungal infections
        Trichinosis, other helminthic infections
    Associated with connective-tissue disease (e.g., sys-
temic lupus erythematosus, rheumatoid arthritis, Sjö-
gren's syndrome)
    Associated with carcinoma
    Idiopathic
Cervical spondylosis
Ankylosing spondylitis
Paget's disease
Pott's disease
Subacute combined degeneration of the spinal cord§
Neurosyphilis (syphilitic meningomyelitis, tabes dorsalis)§
Spinal arachnoiditis (e.g., following subarachnoid hemor-
rhage, meningitis, subarachnoid space injection)§
Chronic epidural infection or granuloma (e.g., tuberculous,
parasitic, fungal)
Electrical or radiation injury of spinal cord
Multiple sclerosis
Syringomyelia‡
Amyotrophic lateral sclerosis‡

Childhood (or Young Adulthood) Onset†
Congenital
    Cerebral spastic diplegia
    Anomalies of spinal cord or vertebrae

Hereditary disease
   Werdnig-Hoffmann disease
   Muscular dystrophies
   Friedreich's ataxia
   Chronic polyneuropathies
   Niemann-Pick disease
   Tay-Sachs disease

Reference
1. General reference 22, p 665, p 960, p 1032.

*Except as noted, all entities may produce paralysis of either legs alone or of all four extremities.
†Usually affects all four extremities.
‡Produces descending paralysis or affects arms first.
§Usually affects legs only.

12-P. Hemiplegia (or Hemiparesis)

Cerebrovascular accident (see 12-N)
   Thrombosis
   Embolism
   Hemorrhage
Transient ischemic attack (TIA)
Migraine syndrome
Head trauma (e.g., brain contusion, subdural or epidural
   hematoma)
Todd's paralysis
Brain tumor (primary or metastatic)
Infection (e.g., brain abscess, encephalitis, subdural em-
   pyema, meningitis)
Nonketotic hyperosmolar coma
Vasculitis
Demyelinating disease (e.g., multiple sclerosis, acute nec-
   rotizing myelitis)
Hereditary disease (e.g., leukodystrophies)
Congenital, perinatal injury

Reference
1. General reference 22, p 37.

12-Q. Peripheral Neuropathy

Primary Motor, Acute (may have sensory involvement)
Guillain-Barré syndrome
Infectious mononucleosis
Viral hepatitis
Porphyria
Diphtheria
Toxins (e.g., organophosphorus compounds, thallium, and vaccine for rabies, typhoid, smallpox)

Sensorimotor, Subacute
Alcoholism with associated nutritional deficiency
Beriberi
Drugs, toxins
  Arsenic
  Mercury
  Thallium
  Lithium
  Gold
  Platinum
  Lead
  Industrial solvents
  Carbon monoxide
  Nitrofurantoin
  Hydralazine
  Phenytoin
  Isoniazid
  Disulfiram
  Amiodarone
Diabetes mellitus
Atherosclerosis
Vasculitis (e.g., polyarteritis nodosa, systemic lupus erythematosus, Wegener's granulomatosis, rheumatoid arthritis)
Sarcoidosis
Subacute asymmetric idiopathic polyneuritis

Sensorimotor, Chronic
Carcinoma
Amyloidosis
Paraproteinemia (especially multiple myeloma, macroglobulinemia, cryoglobulinemia)
Uremia
Beriberi
Alcoholism

Diabetes mellitus
Connective-tissue disease (especially systemic lupus ery-
    thematosus)
Myxedema
Leprosy
Chronic inflammatory polyradiculoneuropathy
Hereditary disease
    Charcot-Marie-Tooth disease
    Déjerine-Sottas disease
    Refsum's disease
    Abetalipoproteinemia
    Metachromatic leukodystrophy
    Roussy-Lévy syndrome
    Fabry's disease
    Familial dysautonomia

Reference
1. General reference 22, p 960.

12-R. Carpal Tunnel Syndrome

Fibrosis or tenosynovitis of flexor tendons
Fracture (e.g., Colles')
Occupational trauma (e.g., jackhammer or typewriter oper-
    ation)
Degenerative arthritis
Wrist ganglion or benign tumor
Pregnancy
Congestive heart failure (with edema)
Amyloidosis
Rheumatoid arthritis
Scleroderma
Systemic lupus erythematosus
Diabetes mellitus
Hypothyroidism
Tuberculosis, other granulomatous diseases (e.g., leprosy,
    sarcoidosis)
Gout
Paget's disease
Acromegaly
Mucopolysaccharidoses

Reference
1. General reference 22.

12-S. Typical Cerebrospinal Fluid Characteristics in Various Diseases

Condition	Pressure (cm H_2O)	WBCs/mm³	Predominant type of WBCs	Glucose (mg/dl)	Protein (mg/dl)	Other
Normal	5–20	<5	100% lymphocytes	50–75% of serum value	<50	Lactate 10–20 mg/dl
Meningitis Bacterial	Usually ↑	100–100,000	85–95% neutrophils	<40, or <40% of blood glucose	45–500	Lactate > 35 mg/dl; ⊕ cultures, Gram's stain, CIE, ELISA
Viral	Normal to ↑	10–500	Lymphocytes (sometimes neutrophils early)	Normal, occasionally ↓	50–200	Lactate < 35 mg/dl

	Pressure	Cells	Cell type	Glucose	Protein	Comments
Tuberculous	↑	50–500	Lymphocytes (occasionally neutrophils)	<40	100–200	Lactate > 35 mg/dl; ⊕ culture &/or Ziehl-Neelsen stain
Fungal (± abscess)	Normal to ↑	25–1000	Lymphocytes	20–40	25–500	Lactate > 35 mg/dl
Neurosyphilis (meningo-vascular or paretic)	Normal to ↑	200–500	Lymphocytes	Normal	40–200	↑ γ-globulins, ⊕ serologic tests (VDRL usually, FTA-ABS "always")
Herpes encephalitis	Normal to ↑	20–500	Lymphocytes	Normal, sometimes →	50–100	↑ RBCs, xanthochromia
Brain abscess*	↑ to ↑↑	20–300 (may be >50,000 if ruptured)	10–80% neutrophils	Normal	75–100	

12-S. Typical Cerebrospinal Fluid Characteristics in Various Diseases (continued)

Condition	Pressure (cm H₂O)	WBCs/mm³	Predominant type of WBCs	Glucose (mg/dl)	Protein (mg/dl)	Other
Neoplasm* Cerebral hemorrhage	Usually ↑ Usually ↑	<100 ↑ in proportion to RBCs (may be 2000–3000)	Lymphocytes Lymphocytes	40–80 Normal, occasionally →	50–1000 ↑ ↑ (<1000)	⊕ cytology ↑ ↑ RBCs, xanthochromia or gross blood
Multiple sclerosis	Normal	<100	Lymphocytes	Normal	<100	↑ γ-globulins (>12% of total protein); ↑ myelin basic protein

*If this diagnosis is suspected, lumbar puncture is contraindicated, at least until after computed tomography has been performed.

References
1. General reference 22.
2. General reference 23.

12-T. Dermatome Chart

Source: Gatz AJ: *Manter's Essentials of Clinical Neuroanatomy and Neurophysiology* (4th ed). Philadelphia: Davis, 1970, p 23.

13 RESPIRATORY SYSTEM

13-A. Cough

Acute
Viral upper respiratory infection
  Pharyngitis
  Rhinitis
  Tracheobronchitis
  Bronchiolitis
  Serous otitis
Bacterial and other infections
  Tracheobronchitis
  Sinusitis, especially maxillary
  Otitis media or externa
  Pneumonia
  Lung abscess
Asthma
Pulmonary edema
Pulmonary embolism
Aspiration pneumonitis
Inhalation of irritants
  Noxious fumes
  Extremely hot or cold air
Foreign body inhalation
Laryngeal inflammation

External or middle ear disease
Acute pleural, pericardial, mediastinal, or diaphragmatic in-
    flammation

Chronic
"Smoker's cough"
Postviral bronchitis
Chronic bronchitis
Chronic rhinosinusitis ("postnasal drip")
Asthma
Neoplasms (especially endobronchial lesions), malignant
    and benign
Bronchiectasis
Lung abscess
Interstitial lung disease (see 13-N)
Recurrent aspiration
    Esophageal reflux
    Hiatus hernia
    Achalasia
Drug-induced
    Beta blockers, selective and nonselective
    Angiotensin-converting enzyme inhibitors
    Amiodarone
Chronic pulmonary edema
Mitral stenosis
Chronic laryngeal inflammation or tumor
Chronic pneumonia, especially tuberculosis and fungal
Cystic fibrosis
External and middle ear disease, chronic
Miscellaneous
    Bronchogenic/mediastinal cyst
    Aortic aneurysm
    Irritation of vagal afferent nerve
        Osteophytes
        Pacemaker wires
    Chronic pleural, pericardial, mediastinal, or diaphrag-
        matic inflammation

Psychogenic

References
1. Irwin RS, Rosen MJ, Braman SS: Cough. *Arch Intern
   Med* 137:1186, 1977.
2. Braman SS, Corrao WM: Cough: Differential Diagnosis
   and Treatment. *Clin Chest Med* 8:177, 1987.
3. Thompson BT, Kazemi H: Pulmonary Problems. In general reference 5, p 168.

13-B. Dyspnea

Acute
Pleuropulmonary causes
  Exacerbation of chronic obstructive lung disease
  Asthma
  Acute tracheobronchitis
  Pneumonitis
  Pulmonary thromboembolism
  Pneumothorax
  Pulmonary edema (see 13-L)
  Pleurisy and/or pleural effusion
  Gastric or other fluid aspiration
  Noxious gas inhalation (including carbon monoxide)
  Upper airway obstruction (see 13-C)
  Collapse of lung segment(s)
  Foreign-body aspiration
  Chest trauma
    Pulmonary contusion
    Rib fractures
    Flail chest
Nonpulmonary causes
  Psychogenic disorders (e.g., anxiety)
  Decreased inspired oxygen tension (e.g., at high altitude)
  Acute neuromuscular dysfunction
  Shock
  Fever
  Increased intracranial pressure
  Metabolic acidosis

Chronic
Pleuropulmonary causes
  Chronic obstructive pulmonary disease
    Chronic bronchitis
    Emphysema
    Cystic fibrosis
  Asthma
  Pulmonary edema or congestion (see 13-L)
  Diffuse interstitial lung disease
  Chronic pneumonia
  Pulmonary vascular disease
    Recurrent pulmonary emboli
    Pulmonary hypertension
    Arteriovenous malformation
  Malignancy
    Bronchogenic carcinoma
    Pulmonary metastatic disease

Respiratory muscle disease
  Phrenic nerve dysfunction
  Neuromuscular disease
    Myasthenia gravis
    Poliomyelitis
    Guillain-Barré syndrome
    Muscular dystrophy
Chest wall abnormalities
Pleural disease
  Effusion
  Fibrothorax
  Primary or metastatic neoplasm
Bronchiectasis
Alveolar filling disease
  Pulmonary alveolar proteinosis
  Alveolar microlithiasis
  Lipoid pneumonia
Lung resection
Upper airway obstruction
Nonpulmonary causes
  Anemia
  Obesity
  Psychogenic disorders
  Ascites
  Metabolic acidosis
  Hyperthyroidism
  Arteriovenous shunt
  Congenital heart disease
  Abnormal hemoglobin

References
1. Ingram RH, Braunwald E: Dyspnea and Pulmonary Edema. In general reference 1, p 141.
2. Thompson BR, Kazemi H: Pulmonary Problems. In general reference 5, p 170.
3. Mahler DA: Dyspnea: Diagnosis and Management. *Clin Chest Med* 8:215, 1987.

13-C. Wheezing

Asthma
Extrinsic
Intrinsic
Exercise- or cold-induced
Drug-induced
   Aspirin
   Beta blockers
   Acetylcysteine
   Indomethacin
   Tartrazine

Wheezing of Other Etiologies
Peripheral airway obstruction
   Bronchitis, chronic or acute
   Bronchiolitis
   Bronchiectasis
   Cystic fibrosis
   Pneumonia
Pulmonary embolism
Cardiac asthma
   Pulmonary edema (see 13-L)
Aspiration
   Foreign body
   Gastric contents
Irritant inhalants
   Toluene diisocyanate
   Sulfur dioxide
Anaphylaxis
Upper airway obstruction
   Extrinsic
      Thyroid enlargement, tumor, hemorrhage
      Lymphoma
      Edema of, or hemorrhage into, subcutaneous tissues
         of neck
      Retropharyngeal edema, hemorrhage, abscess
   Intrinsic
      Epiglottitis
      Foreign body
      Tracheal fracture, stricture, tracheomalacia
      Laryngeal tumor, trauma, edema, spasm
   Functional
Large airway obstruction
   Extrinsic

    Mediastinal hemorrhage or tumor
    Vascular compression
       Aortic aneurysm
       Congenital anomalies
  Intrinsic
    Tracheal stricture, tumor, tracheomalacia
Pulmonary infiltrates with eosinophilia
  Loeffler's syndrome
  Tropical eosinophilia
  Chronic eosinophilic pneumonia
  Bronchopulmonary aspergillosis
  Polyarteritis nodosa
Angioedema
  Idiopathic
  Hereditary angioneurotic edema
Carcinoid syndrome

Reference
1. MacDonnell KF: Differential Diagnosis of Asthma. In
   Weiss EB, Segal MS (Eds): *Bronchial Asthma: Mechanisms and Treatment*. Boston: Little, Brown, 1976, p 679.

13-D. Hemoptysis

Pseudohemoptysis
Blood of upper gastrointestinal origin
Upper airway lesions
  Epistaxis
  Gingival bleeding
  Oropharyngeal carcinoma
  Laryngeal carcinoma or other lesions
  Hereditary hemorrhagic telangiectasia
Serratia marcescens infection

Tracheobronchial Sources
Bronchitis, chronic or acute
Bronchiectasis
Bronchogenic carcinoma
Bronchial adenoma
Foreign body
Endobronchial metastatic neoplasm
Bronchial trauma
Cystic fibrosis
Broncholithiasis
Amyloidosis

Pulmonary Parenchymal Sources
Pneumonia
  Bacterial
  Tuberculous
Pulmonary embolism
Neoplasm
Lung abscess
Fungal infections (especially aspergilloma)
Lung contusion or laceration
Goodpasture's syndrome
Wegener's granulomatosis
Idiopathic pulmonary hemosiderosis
Inhalation injury (toxic gases)
Sequestration
Bronchogenic cyst
Parasitic infestation (e.g., hydatid disease)
Pulmonary endometriosis

Cardiac or Vascular Disorders
Pulmonary edema and congestion
Mitral stenosis
Aortic aneurysm

Primary pulmonary hypertension
Arteriovenous malformation
Eisenmenger's disease
Pulmonary vasculitis
Collagen vascular diseases
Behçet's syndrome
Pulmonary veno-occlusive disease
Pulmonary telangiectasia

Hematologic Disorders
Coagulopathy
  Congenital
  Acquired, including anticoagulant therapy
Thrombocytopenia (see 8-J)

Undiagnosed*

References
1. Tisi GM, Braunwald E: Cough and Hemoptysis. In general reference 1, p 140.
2. Lyons HA: Differential Diagnosis of Hemoptysis and Its Treatment. *Basics RD* 5(2), 1976.

*Five to fifteen percent despite extensive evaluation.

13-E. Cyanosis*

Central Cyanosis
Arterial desaturation
  Decreased inspired oxygen tension
  Pulmonary disease
    Alveolar hypoventilation
    Ventilation-perfusion mismatch
    Impaired oxygen diffusion
  Right-to-left shunt
    Congenital heart disease
    Pulmonary arteriovenous fistulas
    Other intrapulmonary shunts
Hemoglobin abnormalities
  Methemoglobinemia
  Sulfhemoglobinemia
  Hemoglobin with low affinity for oxygen (e.g., hemoglobin Kansas)
Pseudocyanosis
  Polycythemia vera
  Argyria
  Hemochromatosis

Peripheral Cyanosis
Reduced cardiac output
Cold exposure (including Raynaud's phenomenon)
Arterial obstruction
Venous stasis and/or obstruction

References
1. Braunwald E: Cyanosis, Hypoxia, and Polycythemia. In general reference 1, p 145.
2. Guenter CA: Respiratory Function of the Lungs and Blood. In Guenter CA, Welch MA (Eds): *Pulmonary Medicine.* Philadelphia: Lippincott, 1977, p 124.

*Indicates ≥ 5 gm of unsaturated hemoglobin or ≥ 1.5 gm of methemoglobin present.

13-F. Pleuritic Pain*

Chest Wall Disease
Bony thorax
    Costochondritis (Tietze's syndrome)
    Rib fracture or tumor
    Fractured cartilage
    Periostitis
    Periosteal hematoma
    Xiphoidalgia
    Thoracic spondylitis due to arthritis, infection, trauma
Soft tissues
    Muscle spasm (intercostal or pectoral)
    Myositis (see 11-D)
    Fibromyositis
Neural structures
    Intercostal neuritis
    Herpes zoster
    Neurofibromatosis
    Causalgia
    Anterior chest wall syndrome

Pleuropulmonary Disease†
Infectious pleuritis, especially viral
Idiopathic pleurodynia
Pulmonary embolism and infarction
Pneumonia
Pneumothorax
Trauma
Neoplasm
    Primary
    Metastatic
    Direct invasion
Immune-mediated disease, especially:
    Systemic lupus erythematosus
    Postcardiac injury syndrome
    Rheumatoid arthritis
    Vasculitis
Diaphragmatic irritation
    Pancreatitis
    Abscess: subphrenic, splenic, hepatic
Asbestosis
Uremic pleuritis
Radiation pleuritis
Familial polyserositis
Middle lobe syndrome

Mediastinal Disease
Pneumomediastinum
Mediastinitis
Esophageal perforation
Esophageal variceal sclerotherapy
Pericarditis
Tumor, primary or metastatic

References
1. Reich NE, Fremont, RE: *Chest Pain: Systemic Differentiation and Treatment.* New York: Macmillan, 1961.
2. General reference 5, p 224.

*Pleuritic pain is defined as pain accentuated by breathing, coughing, or sneezing.
†Most of the disorders that cause exudative effusions also cause pleuritic pain. See 13-G for a more exhaustive list.

13-G. Pleural Effusion: Exudate

Exudative Pleural Effusion
Infection
  Bacterial
    Empyema
    Parapneumonic effusion
  Tuberculous
  Viral
  Fungal
  Parasitic
  Mycoplasmal
  Rickettsial
Neoplasm
  Direct pleural involvement
    Metastases
    Direct invasion from surrounding structures
    Primary pleural malignancy
  Indirect causes
    Lymphoma
    Ovarian neoplasm (Meigs's syndrome)
Thromboembolic disease
  Pulmonary embolism
  Pulmonary infarction

Immune-mediated diseases
  Rheumatoid disease
  Systemic lupus erythematosus
  Drug-induced lupus
  Wegener's granulomatosis
  Sarcoidosis
  Postcardiac injury syndrome
  Angioimmunoblastic lymphadenopathy
  Sjögren's syndrome
  Progressive systemic sclerosis
Intraabdominal disorders
  Pancreatitis
  Esophageal perforation
  Subphrenic abscess
  Intrahepatic abscess
  Splenic abscess
  Esophageal variceal sclerotherapy
  Postabdominal surgery
  Postpartum state
Drug-induced pleural disease
  Nitrofurantoin
  Methysergide
  Dantrolene
  Bromocriptine
  Procarbazine
  Practolol
  Methotrexate
Inhalation of inorganic dusts
  Asbestosis
Other causes
  Meigs's syndrome
  Yellow nail syndrome
  Uremic pleuritis
  Radiation pleuritis
  Myxedema
  Spontaneous pneumothorax
  Familial Mediterranean fever
  Trapped lung

Hemothorax
Traumatic
  Penetrating or nonpenetrating trauma
  Iatrogenic
Malignancy, especially metastatic
Anticoagulant therapy for pulmonary emboli
Spontaneous
  Secondary to bleeding disorder
  Rupture of intrathoracic vessel or aneurysm

    Ruptured pancreatic pseudocyst
    Thoracic endometriosis
    Idiopathic

Chylothorax
Traumatic
    Penetrating or nonpenetrating trauma
    Surgery
    Iatrogenic
Malignancy
    Lymphoma
    Metastatic malignancy
Idiopathic
Congenital
Pulmonary lymphangiomyomatosis
Pseudochylothorax

References
1. Connors AF, Altose MD: Pleural Disease. In Wolinsky E, Baum GL (Eds): *Textbook of Pulmonary Diseases (3rd ed).* Boston: Little, Brown, (in press).
2. Light RW: *Pleural Diseases.* Philadelphia: Lea & Febiger, 1983.

13-H. Pleural Effusion: Transudate

Cardiac disease
  Congestive heart failure
  Fluid overload
  Constrictive pericarditis
  Obstruction of superior vena cava or azygos vein
Renal disease
  Nephrotic syndrome
  Acute glomerulonephritis
  Urinary tract obstruction
  Peritoneal dialysis
Liver disease
  Cirrhosis with ascites
Thromboembolic disease
  Pulmonary embolism*
Others
  Meigs's syndrome*
  Myxedema*
  Sarcoidosis
  Severe malnutrition (with hypoalbuminemia)
  Iatrogenic (e.g., venous catheter in pleural space)

References
1. Connors AF, Altose MD: Pleural Disease. In Wolinsky E, Baum GL (Eds): *Textbook of Pulmonary Medicine (3rd ed)*. Boston: Little, Brown, (in press).
2. Light RW: *Pleural Diseases*. Philadelphia: Lea & Febiger, 1983.

*Most are exudates.

13-I. Pleural Effusion: Exudate Versus Transudate*

Characteristics of an exudative effusion:
Pleural fluid–serum protein ratio > 0.5
Pleural fluid lactic dehydrogenase (LDH) greater than
two-thirds of the upper limit of normal for serum LDH
Pleural fluid–serum LDH ratio > 0.6.

References
1. Light RW, MacGregor MI, Luchsinger PC, et al: Pleural Effusions: The Diagnostic Separation of Transudates and Exudates. *Ann Intern Med* 77:507, 1972.
2. Light RW: *Pleural Diseases.* Philadelphia: Lea & Febiger, 1983.

*An exudate will have one or more of these three characteristics. A transudate will not have any of these characteristics.

13-J. Empyema

Pulmonary Causes
Pneumonia
Bronchial obstruction
　Tumor
　Foreign body
Hematogenous spread of infection
Bronchopleural fistula
Ruptured abscess
Spontaneous pneumothorax
Bronchiectasis
Rheumatoid disease

Mediastinal Causes
Esophageal fistula
Abscess
　Lymph node
　Osteomyelitis
Pericarditis

Subdiaphragmatic Causes
Abscess (hepatic, pancreatic, splenic, retrogastric)
Peritonitis

Direct Inoculation
Postoperative
  Infected hemothorax
  Leaky bronchial stump (postlobectomy or postpneumo-
    nectomy)
Penetrating chest trauma
  Foreign body in pleural space
Iatrogenic inoculation
  Thoracentesis
  Chest tube

Reference
1. Snider GL, Saleh SS: Empyema of the Thorax in Adults:
Review of 105 Cases. *Chest* 54:410, 1968.

13-K. Pneumothorax

Primary spontaneous pneumothorax
Secondary spontaneous pneumothorax
  Obstructive pulmonary disease
    Chronic airways obstruction
    Asthma
  Malignancy
    Primary lung carcinoma
    Pleural metastatic disease
  Infectious disease
    Lung abscess
    Tuberculosis
  Pulmonary infarction
  Diffuse lung disease
    Idiopathic pulmonary fibrosis
    Eosinophilic granuloma
    Scleroderma
    Rheumatoid disease
    Tuberous sclerosis
    Sarcoidosis
    Lymphangiomyomatosis
    Idiopathic pulmonary hemosiderosis
    Alveolar proteinosis

Pneumoconiosis
  Silicosis
  Berylliosis
Congenital disease
  Cystic fibrosis
  Marfan's syndrome
Catamenial pneumothorax
Neonatal pneumothorax
Traumatic pneumothorax
  Penetrating thoracic trauma
  Barotrauma
  Sudden chest compression
  Iatrogenic

Reference
1. Light RW: *Pleural Diseases.* Philadelphia: Lea & Febiger, 1983, p 187.

13-L. Pulmonary Edema

Elevated Microvascular Pressure
Cardiogenic (see 2-G, under Left Heart Failure)
Volume overload (especially when associated with low
    plasma oncotic pressure)
Neurogenic
  Head trauma
  Intracerebral hemorrhage
  Postictal
Pulmonary venous obstruction
  Chronic mediastinitis
  Anomalous pulmonary venous return
  Congenital pulmonary venous stenosis
  Idiopathic veno-occlusive disease

***Normal Microvascular Pressure (Adult
Respiratory Distress Syndrome)***
Infection
  Sepsis
  Pneumonia
    Bacterial
    Viral
    Mycoplasmal
    Fungal

    Pneumocystis carinii
    Legionnaires' disease
  Miliary tuberculosis
  Toxic shock syndrome
  Malaria
Liquid aspiration
  Gastric contents
  Water (near-drowning)
  Hypertonic contrast media
  Ethyl alcohol
Shock, especially septic (see 2-K)
Multiple trauma and burns
Hematologic disorders
  Diffuse intravascular coagulation
  Transfusion-related leukoagglutinins
  Leukemia
  Unfiltered blood transfusion (controversial)
Inhaled toxic gases
  Oxygen (high concentration)
  Smoke
  Nitrogen dioxide
  Sulfur dioxide
  Chlorine
  Phosgene
  Ozone
  Metallic oxides
  Acid fumes
  Carbon monoxide
  Hydrocarbons
  Cadmium
  Ammonia
Embolism
  Thrombus
  Fat
  Air
  Amniotic fluid
Acute pancreatitis
Drug overdose
  Narcotics
  Propoxyphene
  Chlordiazepoxide
  Aspirin
  Ethchlorvynol
  Barbiturates
  Colchicine
Drug-induced lung injury (see 13-N)
  Paraquat
  Nitrofurantoin

Amiodarone
Immunologic injury
    Goodpasture's syndrome
    Systemic lupus erythematosus
Associated with high negative pleural pressure
    Post-thoracentesis
    Postexpansion of pneumothorax
    Acute bronchial asthma
    Complete upper airway obstruction (e.g., hanging)
Pulmonary lymphatic obstruction
    Fibrotic and inflammatory disease (e.g., silicosis)
    Lymphangitic carcinomatosis
    Post–lung transplant
Miscellaneous
    Acute radiation pneumonitis
    Pulmonary contusion
    Post–cardiopulmonary bypass
    Diabetic ketoacidosis
    Circulating vasoactive substance (e.g., histamine)
    Dextran
    Lymphangiogram dye (mechanism controversial)

Unclear Mechanisms
High-altitude pulmonary edema

References
1. Ingram RH: Adult Respiratory Distress Syndrome. In general reference 1, p 1134.
2. General reference 24, p 1201.
3. Hudson LD: Causes of the Adult Respiratory Distress Syndrome: Clinical Recognition. *Clin Chest Med* 3:195, 1982.

13-M. Respiratory Failure

Central Nervous System Disorders
Drug intoxication
    Sedatives
    Tranquilizers
    Analgesics
    Anesthetics
Vascular disorders, hypoperfusion states
    Intracranial infarction or bleeding (especially brainstem)
    Shock (see 2-K)
Trauma
    Head injury
    Increased intracranial pressure
Infection
    Viral encephalitis
    Bulbar poliomyelitis
Miscellaneous
    Primary alveolar hypoventilation
    Myxedema
    Status epilepticus

Neuromuscular Disorders
Peripheral nerve and anterior horn cell disorders
    Guillain-Barré syndrome
    Poliomyelitis
    Amyotrophic lateral sclerosis
Myoneural junction disorders
    Myasthenia gravis
    Tetanus
    Curare-like drugs
    Anticholinesterase drugs
Muscular disorders
    Polymyositis, dermatomyositis
    Muscular dystrophies
    Myotonia
    Muscle weakness due to, for example, hypophosphatemia, hypokalemia

Chest Wall and Pleural Disorders
Kyphoscoliosis
Chest trauma
    Flail chest
    Multiple rib fractures
    Post-thoracotomy
Pleural disorders
    Large pleural effusions (see 13-G, 13-H)

Tension pneumothorax
Massive fibrosis

Pulmonary Disorders
Airflow limitation, chronic
  Pulmonary emphysema
  Chronic bronchitis
  Asthma, especially status asthmaticus
Airway obstruction, acute
  Foreign body
  Upper airway obstruction (see 13-C)
  Epiglottitis
  Respiratory burns
  Noxious gases
  Bronchospasm, acute (see 13-C)
Alveolar disorders
  Pneumonia
  Aspiration pneumonitis
  Pulmonary edema (see 13-L)
    Elevated microvascular pressure
    Normal microvascular pressure (adult respiratory distress syndrome)
    Combined or unclear mechanisms
Interstitial disorders
  Fibrosing alveolitis
  Interstitial fibrosis and other diffuse disorders (see 13-N)
  Extensive neoplasm
Vascular disorders
  Pulmonary embolus (especially thrombus, fat)
  Obliterative vasculitis
    Primary pulmonary hypertension
    Scleroderma

References
1. Smith JP: Respiratory Failure and Its Management. In Holman CW, Muschenheim C (Eds): *Bronchopulmonary Diseases and Related Disorders.* New York: Harper & Row, 1972, p 694.
2. Pontoppidan H, Geffin B, Lowenstein E: Acute Respiratory Failure. *N Engl J Med* 287:690, 743, 799, 1972.

13-N. Interstitial Lung Disease

Interstitial Disease of Known Etiology
Inorganic dusts
  Silica
  Silicates, especially asbestos, talc, kaolin, diatomaceous
    earth
  Aluminum
    Powdered aluminum
    Bauxite
  Antimony
  Carbon
    Coal
    Granite
  Beryllium
  Mixed dusts
  Metal dusts, especially titanium, tungsten, cadmium
Organic dusts (hypersensitivity pneumonitis)
  Farmer's lung
  Humidifier lung
  Bagassosis
  Many others (see reference 2)
Gases, fumes, vapors, aerosols
  Gases
    Oxygen
    Sulfur dioxide
    Chlorine gas
  Fumes
    Oxides of zinc, cadmium, copper, and others (see ref-
      erence 2)
  Vapors
    Mercury
    Toluene diisocyanate
  Aerosols
    Fats
    Pyrethrum
    Bordeaux mixture
Drugs
  Chemotherapeutic agents
    Busulfan
    Bleomycin
    Cyclophosphamide
    Methotrexate
    Nitrosoureas
    Procarbazine
    Mitomycin
  Antibiotics

      Nitrofurantoin
      Sulfonamides
      Penicillin
    Others
      Diphenylhydantoin
      Drugs causing drug-induced lupus
      Gold salts
      Amiodarone
      Methysergide
      Carbamazepine
      Propranolol
Poisons
  Paraquat
Infections
Radiation injury
Graft-versus-host reaction
Chronic pulmonary edema
Chronic uremia
Adult respiratory distress syndrome (see 13-L)

Interstitial Disease of Unknown Etiology
Idiopathic pulmonary fibrosis
Sarcoidosis
Collagen vascular disease
  Rheumatoid arthritis
  Progressive systemic sclerosis
  Systemic lupus erythematosus
  Polymyositis-dermatomyositis
  Sjögren's syndrome
Vasculitis
  Wegener's granulomatosis
  Lymphomatoid granulomatosis
  Churg-Strauss syndrome
  Hypersensitivity vasculitis
  Overlap syndromes
Eosinophilic lung disease
  Eosinophilic granuloma
  Chronic eosinophilic pneumonia
  Hypereosinophilic syndrome
Idiopathic pulmonary hemosiderosis
Goodpasture's syndrome
Immunoblastic lymphadenopathy
Lymphocytic interstitial pneumonitis
Lymphangiomyomatosis
Amyloidosis
Alveolar proteinosis
Bronchocentric granulomatosis

Inherited disorders
   Familial interstitial fibrosis
   Tuberous sclerosis
   Neurofibromatosis
   Hermansky-Pudlak syndrome
   Niemann-Pick disease
   Gaucher's disease
Liver disease
   Chronic active hepatitis
   Primary biliary cirrhosis
Bowel disease
   Whipple's disease
   Ulcerative colitis
   Crohn's disease
   Weber-Christian disease

References
1. Crystal RG: Interstitial Lung Disorders. In general reference 1, p 1095.
2. Crystal RG, Gadek JE, Ferrans VJ, et al: Interstitial Lung Disease: Current Concepts of Pathogenesis, Staging, and Therapy. *Ann Intern Med* 70:542, 1981.

13-O. Pulmonary Hypertension

Pulmonary Arterial Hypertension (Precapillary)
Vascular disease
  Increased flow
    Patent ductus arteriosus
    Atrial septal defect
      Eisenmenger physiology
    Ventricular septal defect
    Sinus of Valsalva aneurysm
  Decreased flow
    Tetralogy of Fallot
  Primary pulmonary hypertension
  Pulmonary thromboembolic disease
    Thrombotic
    Metastatic neoplasm
    Septic
    Fat
    Foreign material (e.g., talc, mercury)
    Amniotic fluid
    Parasitic (e.g., schistosomiasis)
    Thrombosis due to hemoglobin SS or SC disease
  Pulmonary arteritis
    Raynaud's syndrome
    Scleroderma
    CRST syndrome
    Rheumatoid disease
    Systemic lupus erythematosus
    Polymyositis, dermatomyositis
    Takayasu's arteritis
    Granulomatous arteritis
Lung and pleural disease
  Emphysema
  Diffuse interstitial or alveolar disease (see 13-N)
    Sarcoidosis
    Other granulomatous diseases
    Interstitial fibrosis
    Neoplasm
      Metastatic
      Alveolar cell carcinoma
    Bronchiectasis
    Alveolar microlithiasis
    Alveolar proteinosis
    Idiopathic hemosiderosis
    Cystic fibrosis
    Post–lung resection

Pleural disease
  Fibrothorax
Chest deformity
  Kyphoscoliosis
  Thoracoplasty
  Poliomyelitis
  Muscular dystrophy
Alveolar hypoventilation
  Neuromuscular (see 11-D)
  Obesity
  Primary alveolar hypoventilation
  Sleep apnea syndrome
  Chronic upper airway obstruction in children
High-altitude pulmonary hypertension

Pulmonary Venous Hypertension (Postcapillary)
Cardiac disease
  Left ventricular failure (see 2-G)
  Mitral valve disease
    Mitral stenosis
    Mitral insufficiency
  Left atrial obstruction
    Myxoma or other tumor
    Supravalvular stenotic ring
    Thrombus
  Cor triatriatum
Pulmonary venous disease
  Medastinal neoplasm or granuloma
  Mediastinitis
  Anomalous pulmonary venous return
  Congenital pulmonary venous stenosis
  Idiopathic pulmonary veno-occlusive disease

References
1. General reference 24, p 1203.
2. Fowler NO: Pulmonary Hypertension. In Baum GE (Ed): *Textbook of Pulmonary Diseases (2nd ed).* Boston: Little, Brown, 1974, p 701.
3. Moser KM (Ed): *Pulmonary Vascular Diseases.* New York: Marcel Dekker, 1979.

13-P. Mediastinal Masses by Predominant Compartment

Anterior
Substernal thyroid
Thymoma
Lymphoma
Germinal cell neoplasm (e.g., dermoid)
Ascending aortic aneurysm
Parathyroid tumor
Mesenchymal neoplasm (e.g., lipoma or fibroma)
Hematoma
Bronchogenic cyst

Middle
Lymphoma
Metastatic neoplasm (pulmonary or extrapulmonary)
Sarcoid lymphadenopathy
Infectious granulomatous disease
Bronchogenic cyst
Vascular dilatation
   Superior vena cava
   Azygos vein
   Pulmonary artery
Aortic arch aneurysm
Vascular anomaly
Pleuropericardial cyst
Lymph node hyperplasia
Mononucleosis-associated adenopathy
Primary or tracheal neoplasm
Hematoma

Anterior Cardiophrenic Angle
Pleuropericardial cyst or tumor
Foramen of Morgagni hernia
Fat pad
Diaphragmatic lymph node enlargement (e.g., lymphoma)
Pulmonary parenchymal mass
Cardiac aneurysm
Pericardial fat necrosis

Posterior
Neurogenic tumor
Meningocele
Esophageal lesion
   Neoplasm

Diverticulum
Megaesophagus of any etiology (e.g., achalasia)
Hiatus hernia
Bochdalek hernia
Thoracic spine lesion
  Neoplasm
  Infectious spondylitis
  Fracture with hematoma
Extramedullary hematopoiesis
Descending aortic aneurysm
Mediastinal abscess
Pancreatic pseudocyst
Lymph node hyperplasia
Hematoma
Cystic lesion
  Neurenteric cyst
  Gastroenteric cyst
  Thoracic duct
  Bronchogenic cyst

Diffuse Mediastinal Widening
Bronchogenic carcinoma
Mediastinal hemorrhage
Granulomatous mediastinitis
  Idiopathic
  Tuberculosis
  Histoplasmosis
Mediastinal lipomatosis
Pneumomediastinum
Acute mediastinitis

References
1. General reference 24, p 2314.
2. Wychulis AR, Payne WS, Clagett OT, et al: Surgical
   Treatment of Mediastinal Tumors: A 40 Year Experience.
   J Thorac Cardiovasc Surg 62: 379, 1971.

13-Q. Solitary Pulmonary Nodule

Neoplasm
  Bronchogenic carcinoma
  Metastatic malignancy
  Hamartoma
  Bronchial adenoma
  Lymphoma
  Plasmacytoma
  Amyloidosis
  Other rare neoplasms
Infection
  Tuberculosis
  Histoplasmosis
  Aspergillosis (mucoid impaction)
  Cryptococcosis
  Dirofilaria immitis
Immune disorders
  Rheumatoid nodule
  Wegener's granulomatosis
Developmental disorders
  Bronchogenic cyst
  Arteriovenous fistula
  Sequestration
  Varicose pulmonary vein
  Bronchial atresia
Other
  Pulmonary infarction
  Lipoid pneumonia
  Hematoma

Reference
1. General reference 24, p 2170.

13-R. Solitary Pulmonary Nodule: Distinguishing Benign From Malignant Lesions

	Benign	Malignant
CLINICAL FINDINGS		
Age*	<35	>40
Symptoms	Absent	Present
History	Tuberculosis exposure	Smoker
	Histoplasmosis exposure	Extrathoracic
	Nonsmoker	malignancy
	Mineral oil use	Prior
		malignancy
X-RAY FINDINGS		
Size	<2 cm	>2 cm
Border	Smooth, well-defined	Ill-defined, lobulated
Calcification*	Laminated, "popcorn," or multiple punctate	Eccentric if present
Doubling time*	<1 or >18 months	1–18 months

*These factors are most important in distinguishing benign from malignant lesions.
Source: Modified from Fraser RG, Paré JAP (Eds). *Diagnosis of Diseases of the Chest* (2nd ed.). Philadelphia: Saunders, 1978, p 2073.

13-S. Elevated Hemidiaphragm

Pseudoelevation
Subpulmonic effusion
Diaphragmatic neoplasm

True Elevation
Intrathoracic conditions
  Lobar or segmental atelectasis
  Pneumonia
  Pulmonary infarction
  Rib fracture
  Pleurisy
Paralysis or paresis due to phrenic nerve dysfunction
  Bronchogenic carcinoma or mediastinal malignancy
  Surgical or nonsurgical trauma
  Neurologic disorders
    Myelitis
    Encephalitis
    Herpes zoster
    Poliomyelitis
    Myotonia
    Serum sickness following tetanus antitoxin
    Diphtheria
  Extrinsic pressure
    Substernal thyroid
    Aortic aneurysm
  Infection
    Tuberculosis
    Pneumonia
    Empyema or pleuritis
    Infection of the neck or cervical spine
  Radiation therapy
  Idiopathic
Intraabdominal pathology
  Subphrenic or hepatic abscess
  Pancreatitis
  Other intrahepatic mass lesion, especially malignancy
  Other intraabdominal mass
  Splenic infarct
Eventration
Traumatic rupture of the diaphragm

References
1. Riley EA: Idiopathic Diaphragmatic Paralysis. *Am J Med* 32:404, 1962.

2. General reference 24, p 1871.
3. Felson B: *Chest Radiology.* Philadelphia: Saunders, 1973, p 421.

13-T. Factors Associated with an Increased Risk of Postoperative Pulmonary Complications

General factors
    Cigarette smoking (especially > 10 pack-years)
    Chronic bronchitis
    Obesity
    Age > 70 years
    Concomitant illness
    Alcohol abuse
Surgical factors
    Thoracic surgery (especially with resection of functional lung)
    Upper abdominal surgery
Pulmonary function
    Forced vital capacity (FVC) < 70% of predicted
    Forced expiratory volume in 1 second (FEV_1) < 70% of predicted
    FEV_1/FVC < 65%
    Forced expiratory flow from 25–75% of FVC (FEF_{25-75}) < 50% of predicted
    Maximum voluntary ventilation (MVV) < 50% of predicted
    Diffusing capacity of carbon monoxide (DL_{CO}) < 50% of predicted
Arterial blood gases
    PCO_2 > 45 mm Hg
    Hypoxemia not a reliable indicator

References
1. Gass GD, Olsen GN: Preoperative Pulmonary Function Testing to Predict Post-operative Morbidity and Mortality. *Chest* 89:127, 1986.
2. Tisi G: State of the Art: Preoperative Evaluation of Pulmonary Function. *Am Rev Respir Dis* 119:295, 1979.
3. Bendixen HH: Pulmonary Problems in the Postoperative Patient. In Fishman AP (Ed): *Pulmonary Diseases and Disorders.* New York: McGraw-Hill, 1980, p 1716.

GENERAL REFERENCES

1. Braunwald E, Isselbacher KJ, Petersdorf RG, et al (Eds): *Harrison's Principles of Internal Medicine* (11th ed). New York: McGraw-Hill, 1987.
2. Orland MJ, Saltman RJ (Eds): *Manual of Medical Therapeutics* (25th ed). Boston: Little, Brown, 1986.
3. Friedman HH (Ed): *Problem-Oriented Medical Diagnosis* (3rd ed). Boston: Little, Brown, 1983.
4. DeGowin EL, DeGowin RL: *Bedside Diagnostic Examination* (5th ed). New York: Macmillan, 1987.
5. Samiy AH, Douglas RG, Barondess JA (Eds): *Textbook of Diagnostic Medicine.* Philadelphia: Lea & Febiger, 1987.

Acid-Base and Electrolyte Disorders
6. Maxwell MH, Kleeman CR, Narins RG (Eds): *Clinical Disorders of Fluid and Electrolyte Metabolism* (4th ed). New York: McGraw-Hill, 1987.

Cardiovascular System
7. Braunwald E (Ed): *Heart Disease* (3rd ed). Philadelphia: Saunders, 1988.

Endocrine/Metabolic System

8. Felig P, Baxter JD, Broadus AE, Frohman LA (Eds): *Endocrinology and Metabolism* (2nd ed). New York: McGraw-Hill, 1987.
9. Williams RH (Ed): *Textbook of Endocrinology* (7th ed). Philadelphia: Saunders, 1985.

Eye

10. Newell FW: *Ophthalmology: Principles and Concepts* (6th ed). St. Louis: Mosby, 1986.
11. Scheie HG, Albert DM: *Textbook of Ophthalmology* (9th ed). Philadelphia: Saunders, 1977.

Gastrointestinal and Hepatic Systems

12. Sleisenger MH, Fordtran JS (Eds): *Gastrointestinal Disease: Pathophysiology, Diagnosis, Management* (3rd ed). Philadelphia: Saunders, 1983.
13. Eastwood GL (Ed): *Core Textbook of Gastroenterology.* Philadelphia: Lippincott, 1984.
14. Zakim D, Boyer TD (Eds): *Hepatology: A Textbook of Liver Disease.* Philadelphia: Saunders, 1982.

Genitourinary System

15. Brenner BM, Rector FC (Eds): *The Kidney* (3rd ed). Philadelphia: Saunders, 1986.
16. Schrier RW (Ed): *Renal and Electrolyte Disorders* (3rd ed). Boston: Little, Brown, 1986.

Hematologic System

17. Wintrobe MM, Lee GR, Boggs DR, et al (Eds): *Clinical Hematology* (8th ed). Philadelphia: Lea & Febiger, 1981.
18. Williams WJ, Beutler E, Erslev AJ, Lichtman MA: *Hematology* (3rd ed). New York: McGraw-Hill, 1983.

Infectious Disease

19. Hoeprich PD (Ed): *Infectious Diseases* (3rd ed). Philadelphia: Harper & Row, 1983.

Integument

20. Fitzpatrick TB, Eisen AZ, Wolff K, et al (Eds): *Dermatology in General Medicine* (3rd ed). New York: McGraw-Hill, 1987.

Musculoskeletal System

21. Kelley WN, Harris ED, Ruddy S, Sledge CB (Eds): *Textbook of Rheumatology* (2nd ed). Philadelphia: Saunders, 1985.

Nervous System
22. Adams RD, Victor M: *Principles of Neurology* (3rd ed).
    New York: McGraw-Hill, 1985.
23. Baker AB, Joynt RJ (Eds): *Clinical Neurology* (2nd ed).
    New York: Harper & Row, 1986.

Respiratory System
24. Fraser RG, Paré JAP (Eds): *Diagnosis of Diseases of
    the Chest* (2nd ed). Philadelphia: Saunders, 1978.

INDEX